Praise for
Feng Shui Chic

"If you trust that feng shui can be applied to both micro and macro spaces and objects, it's no stretch to see the importance of overlaying this system onto personal style. The connected body, mind, spirit, and fashion wisdom in this book is definitely worth exploring."
—Karen Rauch Carter, author of the bestselling *Move Your Stuff, Change Your Life*

"*Feng Shui Chic* provides an interesting and provocative approach to the link between our external environment, our bodies, and how we adorn them to achieve a sense of being centered."
—Master Angi Ma Wong, celebrity feng shui consultant and bestselling author of *Feng Shui Dos and Taboos* and *Feng Shui Dos and Taboos for Love*

"*Feng Shui Chic* is a fun book. Honoring and nurturing ourselves is the true essence of life, and Meltzer and Andrusia have fun showing you ways to do just that. Feng shui is about how easily we flow through and with life—how our world affects how much energy we have and how we feel. This book covers myriad ways to support your overall health and well-being."
—Sally Fretwell, feng shui consultant and author of *Feng Shui: Back to Balance.*

"Meltzer and Andrusia has successfully elevated feng shui to a new level. The information is both inspirational and practical. Anyone who wants to improve any or all aspects of their life needs to read this book! It can change your life while giving you balance and a fresh perspective."
—Rick Haskins, executive vice president, Lifetime Television for Women

"Carole Meltzer's application of feng shui in my wardrobe has helped me in ways I never imagined. Her advice on fashion and color has made me not only feel better but perform better at everything I do. In addition, whenever I take Carole's fashion advice, I get countless compliments. Given the fact that I am seen by millions on TV every day because of my job, how I look is very important. I wouldn't trust just anyone, but I trust Carole completely."
—Julie Chen, news anchor of *The Early Show* on CBS and host of the CBS reality show *Big Brother*

2003

To Susia,
"Keep Truckin'"
Blessings,
Carole

Feng Shui

Chic

Change Your Life with Spirit and Style

Feng Shui Master Carole Swann Meltzer, B.T.B., and David Andrusia, A.B., M.A.

A Fireside Book

Published by Simon & Schuster

New York   London   Toronto   Sydney   Singapore

This publication contains the opinions and ideas of its author. It is intended to provide helpful and informative material on the subjects addressed in the publication. It is sold with the understanding that the author and publisher are not engaged in rendering medical, health, psychological, or any other kind of personal professional services in the book. If the reader requires personal medical, health, or other assistance or advice, a competent professional should be consulted.

The author and publisher specifically disclaim all responsibility for any liability, loss, or risk, personal or otherwise, that is incurred as a consequence, directly or indirectly, of the use and application of any of the contents of this book.

FIRESIDE
Rockefeller Center
1230 Avenue of the Americas
New York, NY 10020

Copyright © 2003 by Carole Meltzer

FIRESIDE and colophon are registered trademarks
of Simon & Schuster, Inc.

For information regarding special discounts for bulk purchases,
please contact Simon & Schuster Special Sales
at 1-800-456-6798 or business@simonandschuster.com

Designed by Diane Hobbing of SNAP-HAUS GRAPHICS

Manufactured in the United States of America

1   2   3   4   5   6   7   8   9   10

Library of Congress Cataloging-in-Publication Data
Meltzer, Carole Swann.
Feng shui chic : change your life with spirit and style /
Carole Swann Meltzer and David Andrusia.
p.   cm.
"A Fireside book."
Includes bibliographical references and index.
1. Feng shui. I. Andrusia, David. II. Title.
BF1779.F4 M45   2003
133.3'337—dc21   2002027870

ISBN 0-7432-2196-6

To save a memory of the ancients is noble.

Ever since I first traveled to Hong Kong, I have been enthralled by the stories of the Chinese ancestors and their heritage. As I matured and had children of my own, I began to feel the importance of heritage and the necessity of discovering and cherishing one's roots.

Although I am an American, I was asked by my master before me to preserve what was considered his cultural heritage. Ever since then, I have taken it upon myself to go step by step, and I have written this book based on past dynasties, which were recorded as the Chou manuscripts. In the process, I have adapted these ancient traditions in order to meet today's lifestyles.

I have dedicated this book to you, with love in my heart. Thank you, Grand Master Leung, for your inspiration and encouragement, for the gift of this living legacy. Your memory and your exceptional spirit, with insight and details for living, are as vibrant as an artist's palette and as colorful for the life we are given. I am most privileged to have received this rich tradition, weaving the most beautiful tapestry of cultural customers and lifestyle strategies, to experience happiness with the joy of living, and to share it with others.

Carole Meltzer

I do not claim to be an accomplished writer. However, every written word is a simple explanation that has been retained through translation. The facts have been given to David Andrusia, a most gifted writer, and have been interpreted and organized while capturing the authenticity and teachings of feng shui.

As previously mentioned in my dedication, my main purpose in writing this book is to leave a living heritage to those seeking knowledge for a harmonious life. I am most grateful to the following people who have enriched and shared my journey.

A big thanks to David Andrusia for your constant assistance, knowledgeable input, and support. You have taken the past and created present-perfect prose.

My deepest gratitude to Marcela Landres, whose insight and inspiration have made my dream a reality. Your skill and passion to develop *Feng Shui Chic* cannot be overstated. With deep respect, I thank you with all my heart, for your continuous vision.

Great gratitude to Madeleine Morel, the dearest book agent, whose time and devotion helped find the perfect publisher for this book.

I must give credit to all the souls and spirits at Simon & Schuster for their continuous encouragement and knowledge in helping to create this book.

To all my clients and to their spirit guides, I am most grateful to have been a part of touching their lives as they have touched mine. To Jason, your outward quest in seeking knowledge and growth has created paths to do so. Thank you, Sam, for your knowledge and teachings of voice for communication. In appreciation to Neiman Marcus, whose support of artisans and my creative visions make the difference! Thank you for being part of my family.

I am most grateful to Master Lin Yun and Grand Master Leung of Compass School for their teachings and blessings. In deep appreciation to the following organizations: Dancers in Transition—your spirit and grace balance and bridge life through theater. ASID—your creative energy makes the world a more beautiful place. Thank you, fellow feng shui experts, for lighting the path of healing; you know who you are. Thank you to coach Judy for fitness on the run.

To my dear friend Steven Crowler, whose artistry and drawings give life to this text through illustration.

I feel most fortunate for the friendships I have developed along the way. To the Mountain Mamas—we are so lucky! Thank you to Jodi, Felissa, Dezia for your truths, sounds, and healings, which have helped enrich my path. To Debbie who creates order out of chaos with a smile—I couldn't have written *Feng Shui Chic* without you.

I thank the following artists who have shared their wisdom and vision with me, and the world. In deep respect for your friendship and inspiration: Erté, Ken Noland, Andy Warhol, and Hans Erni.

In devotion to my mother and bubbie, whose teachings of love gave me early encouragement to call on spirit and follow my star. To my marriage mom, thank you for your wisdom and love.

I am most fortunate for the gifts of love my family have consistently given to me. Thank you to my daughters, Jori, Lani, and Tara—your unconditional love and support offered daily are my wellness spring, replenishing and nurturing my soul. To my son, Jon, and grandsons, Shane and Connor, your laughter is joy.

In devotion to my husband, Peter, you are my "anchor in the

storm." I am most grateful for the road we have traveled together, which has opened possibilities for us to seek and grow with love.

To my readers and the spirit with you, thank you. Blessings and love.

David Andrusia

A thousand thanks and fantastic feng shui to
- Carole Meltzer, for your enormous expertise, extreme encouragement, and endless energy. We've created a book from our hearts, and that's the very best kind. Here's to the first of many!
- Marcela Landres, editor extraordinaire, for your nonstop support, unwavering belief in *Feng Shui Chic*, and kind words always. I promise that one day I will be able to conjugate the past subjunctive in Spanish. *¡Muchissimas gracias por todo!*
- Madeleine Morel, awesome agent, fine friend, expert on all things English, constant source of amusement—and Platonic scholar of note. Your A in "CC" is duly noted!
- Kate Lapin, copyeditor of unparalleled kindness and wisdom. A big kiss to you!
- my friends Karen, Robin, Mike, Wolfgang, Raegan, Greg, Rick, and Doug, without whose lifesaving laptop and "you can do its!" there would be no *Feng Shui Chic*.

CONTENTS

Feng Shui
Chic

What Is Feng Shui Chic?

Feng Shui Chic. As I look at these three words, I can't help but smile. After all, the very word *chic* implies all that is trendy and new. And while I am the biggest devotee of feng shui anywhere, it's hard to think of this ancient practice as trendy or chic!

Yet that, my friends, is exactly what this book is about: Feng Shui Chic. This is because what we wear, how we dress, our makeup, and even the scent we wear influences our energy, and thus whole aspects of our lives. It's about looking and feeling your absolute finest through the principles of feng shui—not sometimes, not once in a while, but for every day of your life.

The Practice of Feng Shui Chic

About ten years ago, after moving back to the States following many years in Asia, I began to incorporate Feng Shui Chic into the traditional feng shui I was performing—and the results of this combination were fruitful indeed. I believed I had touched upon a winning synthesis of personal and spatial feng shui.

Feng Shui Chic is based on the study and practice of Chinese aesthetic medicine. Used for centuries, this practice combines medicine with aesthetics.

Why? Because in Asia, psychological and physical health are seen as one and the same, not as two distinct, unrelated forces. In fact, beauty—seen as somewhat superficial to Western minds—is a function of body alignment. And if you know just a bit about Chinese medicine and body meridians, you know that body alignment is seen as a form of preventive medicine—the first step to beauty inside and out.

A large part of this book is about achieving wellness through internal, as well as external, health. By balancing energy, we balance our internal organs in conjunction with spatial alignment.

While pondering the various uses of feng shui, it struck me: In modern society, we feng shui our houses, our offices, our apartments. But, unlike many people in Eastern cultures, we don't feng shui ourselves.

Feng shui, after all, isn't merely about moving a piece of furniture. If it were, we'd all be as rich as Anna Nicole Smith, as skinny as Courteney Cox Arquette, and as professionally successful as Carly Fiorentina, the head of Hewlett-Packard.

Sometimes, the best ideas are those that are staring you in the face. Why hadn't I, a fashionista from the word go, thought about this earlier?

And then I wondered: How come

- a chic scarf can look so Audrey Hepburn–like in some circumstances, and so pretentious and showy in others?
- a form-fitting skirt can set the world on fire in some settings, and just look slutty on other occasions?
- a boxy suit can invest you with authority in key situations, and do nothing for you at other times?

And thus the notion of Feng Shui Chic was born.

After coming to this conclusion about the missing adoption of personal feng shui for American audiences, I began working with friends, family, and private clients. Today, after years of modification and change, I can say with certitude that using this system—

the steps of Feng Shui Chic—will let you have the power and passion you so richly deserve in all aspects of your life.

What This Book Will Do for You

But that's just the start! While looking wonderful—and of course, superstylish—is certainly a goal we all share, there's much more to this book than that. Because by using the guidelines of *Feng Shui Chic,* you can change not only your dress and appearance, but many other aspects of your life. In so doing, you can attract a whole new range of opportunities to you.

Sound too good to be true? I assure you, new friends, that it isn't. I know that this system works because I have seen its results in the thousands of women—clients and friends alike—with whom I have worked over the past twenty years.

This is the start of a whole new way of living for you. In a phrase, it is the beginning of a life of Feng Shui Chic.

Have you ever wondered how some people seem to flow effortlessly through life, achieving their heart's desires and then some? And how, conversely, others among us face a series of roadblocks so daunting that we sometimes wonder how to make it through yet another day?

We speak, don't we, of "golden girls" or of "the boys of summer," those women and men who seem to have it all from the day they were born. While there's no denying the powers of circumstance and fate, it is equally true that we can chart our own destiny if only we know how. Gaining this power in order to make the most of your life is what this book is all about.

In *Feng Shui Chic,* I will teach you how to use the time-tested fundamentals of feng shui to
- advance your career
- improve relationships with your loved ones and friends
- attract money

- gain wisdom and inner strength
- tap into your sensual energy

And, most important of all, how to

- find the love you so richly deserve . . .

. . . all while looking more chic than you ever dreamed you could.

Sound too good to be true? Odd? Impossible to achieve? At first blush, perhaps it does. But I assure you—and I say this only from years of experience—that all of the above are possible when using the easy-to-follow program of Feng Shui Chic. More than anything, this book is about finding personal power and harnessing its force to gain the best out of your life . . . today, tomorrow, and in the times to come.

"But how is this possible?" you may well ask. To know the answer to this question, you must first know more about the ancient practice of feng shui . . . and telling people how to change their lives through feng shui is what I like to do more than anything else.

In the following chapter through chapter five, I will provide you with the basics of feng shui, with a special focus on how you can adapt these ancient traditions to your daily modern life. Once you have this understanding, I'll be able to show you how chi energy can interact with your body, fashion, color, and scent to maximize life opportunities . . . and how you can achieve balance in all aspects of your life. In this way, you will have a potent formula for change—and be able to achieve personal enrichment of the most satisfying kind.

Of course, if you are eager to find a Feng Shui Chic solution to a pressing problem, you may go straight to the appropriate chapter now—e.g., chapter six for love, chapter seven for career. How can you do this? Because when you have a headache, you take an aspirin with complete confidence that it will lessen your pain, even though you may not be able to explain precisely how or why it works.

Similarly, while it is best to have a basic understanding of the principles of Feng Shui Chic, you can use this system with complete confidence that it will solve almost any problem—without your needing to know the whys and wherefores as fully as a feng shui master does, and looking your best while you do.

Does Feng Shui Really Work?

I've always felt that one reason the very real benefits of feng shui have been derided in some circles is that the critical parties do not understand the true nature and background of this ancient art. To be perfectly fair, I can understand their concerns, because many Western practitioners use a form of feng shui that is but a weak dilution of its Asian origins.

For now, I'd like to dispel the commonly held notions about feng shui. It is absolutely not about

- changing the furniture in your home or office to make a million dollars
- using one fixed color as a good luck talisman
- repositioning mirrors to cast the evil eye on your enemies

And now for my personal favorite—it is certainly not about

- witchcraft or religion

Most important of all, it is vital to recognize one fact: Feng shui is not a quick fix, an easy answer, or a one-time solution. It is an ongoing practice, one that changes with the season, with your immediate goals, and with your situation in life. Far from being the stagnant concept some Western writers have described, feng shui is as flowing and as constantly changing as life itself.

Know this: I am not advocating that you blindly let feng shui dictate what you do in any aspect of your life. Far from it, as feng shui (and let's correct another misconception) is about letting you take an active role in the direction of your life. In a nutshell: We can use feng shui's principles to work for us, and that is what you'll learn to do here.

All this will become apparent when we get into the chapters dealing with the nine zones, or life areas, which begin on page 72. For now, this is what you should know: "Where am I going?" and "What do I intend to do/achieve?" are the mantras that are the primary focus of this book . . . and the ones you should repeat to yourself every day of your life.

Is Feng Shui Chic About Color?

Frankly, Feng Shui Chic is not merely about what color or cut of clothes to wear. Nor is it a traditional wardrobe guide. It is, however, about using style to achieve your goals and dreams—and look absolutely fabulous as you do.

Interestingly, this is something Asians have always known: how to align with the season in order to balance oneself with the environment . . . and how to attract the very best from all the richness that exists in the outside world.

At this point, I know you're eager for an example. Hold on, honeys—and let's look at precisely how this works.

In the warm seasons, for instance, we need to balance the external temperature with water energy, which cools us down by optimizing our chi. We do this by wearing more blue, green, and black. At the same time, wearing unstructured clothes helps us balance the heat of the day. Conversely, in winter, we need to add fire elements to our wardrobe, with red the best color choice. In this season, structured clothing helps keep us warm from the raw elements outside.

It is fascinating to me—and I think it will be to you, too—how we have incorporated many of these ideas into our contemporary North American way of dressing. For instance, we

- don't wear white after Labor Day (remember what happened to Patricia Hearst when she wore white shoes in the fall in the movie *Serial Mom?*)

- wear black while mourning
- may choose to wear bright colors to change a blue mood

Of course, these notions represent a mixed bag. Some are traditional, others more in line with Feng Shui Chic. But all have this in common: They show how we use color to suit a season or mood, just as Asians have done for centuries on end. How did they do this? In China, folk went so far as to color their clothes with the plants of the season, using bark, berries, and grasses to be in touch with nature in a very visceral way.

Here's the best part: In the zone chapters coming up soon, you'll learn how to do so scientifically, based on the Chou Silk manuscripts that have only recently been discovered by Western eyes. This is because the Chou Silk manuscripts contain the most complete information ever recorded on how the ancients used color, season, and cycles to manage many aspects of their lives, from agriculture to social interaction.

In many ways, the concept of Feng Shui Chic is based on my knowledge of these manuscripts, which align color with season more intricately than, until recently, had ever been known in the West. My system is based on these ancient texts—the first program ever crafted for modern readers in America and beyond.

The Origins of Feng Shui Chic

Since the earliest times, the way people dressed in China spoke volumes about who they were and their station in life. For instance, Grand Emperor Huang Ti was the only person in all of China who was allowed to wear the color yellow, because this color was assigned exclusively to royalty; but the caste implications of this lore tell us only half the tale. (If I were empress, forget yellow—I'd be the only one allowed to wear Prada. But that's another story.)

Equally important is that yellow also signified the so-called "mandate of heaven," and it announced the grand emperor as the

"Heavenly Ruler." In ancient China, rulers were so omnipotent that they were loath to separate themselves from the divine powers from which they declared themselves descendants.

During the "dog days of summer," Grand Emperor Huang Ti lived in a singular residence known as the Temple of Ancestors and wore his traditional yellow. This color not only bespoke his imperial roots, but was deemed, in the pages of the old Chinese Almanac, to be good feng shui as well. Interestingly, feng shui also dictated Huang Ti's food choices.

As autumn drew near, the emperor moved to three Western Palaces. In this location, he wore white, a color associated with the harvest. He ate dog (as is still done in some Asian lands) and sesame, as dictated by feng shui.

When winter arrived, the emperor moved to the Northern Palace. He wore black garments as per his element sign and time of year.

How were the grand emperor's colors and foods chosen? By his element sign, as determined by the date of his birth. Each element—wood, earth, water, fire, and metal—thus corresponds to a specific personality type and informs your feng shui colors as well. As we soon shall see, these change both with the season and with the time of day (or night).

Just as the emperor ensured his good health, expanded his wealth, and achieved peace in his personal life through feng shui, so, too, will you. That is the basis of Feng Shui Chic.

How important was the use of color in dress back then? Proof positive is this: Anyone who dared to wear the emperor-only yellow was immediately put to death. Suffice it to say that personal feng shui was considered a matter of no small consequence among the ancient Chinese!

In ancient Asia, then, one's social position and caste had everything to do with the colors one could wear. Happily, today we can use the concepts of Feng Shui Chic without fear of censure or bodily harm. What this means: We, too, can empower ourselves with the force of any emperor's new clothes. (In our times, we do have the "fashion police"; thank God their only weapons are words!)

The Contemporary Uses of Color

The present uses of color are not so terribly different from those the emperor used, although—thankfully—we tend to wear colors symbolically rather than imperially or magisterially. Just consider how
- brides wear white
- judges sport black
- soldiers wear camouflage green
- fashionistas wear the colors of the season (and true divas *never* wear the same thing twice)

In the first two cases, especially, these color choices have sprung not from whim, but from carefully orchestrated (and evolving) social patterns. As such, they provide a social, as well as cultural, context for how and why we wear color at different times in our lives.

Why Is Feng Shui Chic Important?

Literally, *feng shui* translates as "wind and water." Its greater meaning, however, is more metaphorical. In its deepest form, feng shui has to do with the flow and balance of natural energies, all of which lie between the boundaries of water and wind. In fact, the fullest, most complete use of feng shui is in the blending and unifying of these two forces. By so doing, we bring nature and humankind into balance. We also achieve the sense of harmony that is requisite to achieving inner peace . . . and this sets the stage on which to reach our goals.

What is the significance of water and wind? Water and wind show movement and change in nature. Their combination creates vapor or breath, the very essence of life.

In this book, I present for the first time the specific principles and color directions that the ancients used. This is a system of order founded in predynastic China and is still followed in many parts of Asia today.

From What Sources Does Feng Shui Chic Spring?

The body bagua chart, which you'll soon see on the following pages, is based on an ancient text that has only recently been presented in the West. I have spent countless hours examining the translations of the Chou Silk manuscripts, which date from 300 B.C., and which are now on exhibit in the Arthur Sackler Foundation in Washington, D.C.

What, exactly, is the body bagua? It is a system based on Chinese aesthetic medicine. In a later chapter, I will explain this concept in full, but for now you can think of the body bagua as a feng shui placement chart for the body. According to the body bagua, certain body parts align with what the Chinese call guas—or what I call life zones. These zones reflect life areas, such as wealth, fame, and love. The chart tells the story in visual terms.

The Chou Silk manuscripts are extraordinary in many ways. I was especially struck by the representations of the seasons that an early calendar includes. In each season, we see the five elements—earth, water, wood, metal, and fire—and corresponding colors. These fascinating manuscripts show, above all else, how the season, elements, and colors connect with nature to manifest energy flow. What this means is that we can manipulate color to balance our energy and reach our goals in life.

Just as the ancients did, you, too, will learn how to use your feng shui colors to counteract negativity and ensure a successful outcome in all areas of your life. But first, let's learn more about feng shui itself before delving deeper into the subject of Feng Shui Chic. And that's precisely what we'll do in the next chapter; come there with me now.

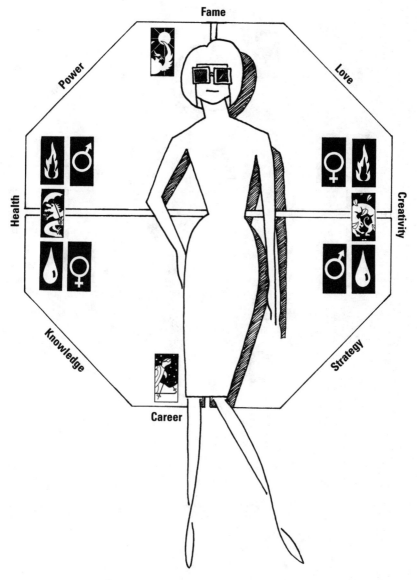

The Body Bagua, Front

What Is Feng Shui Chic? | 11

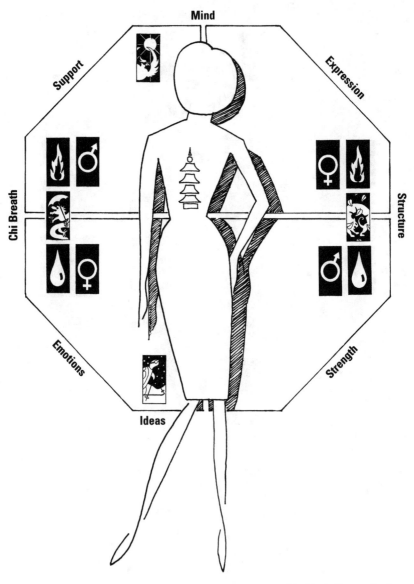

The Body Bagua, Back

What Is Feng Shui?

In chapter one, I shared with you some popular misconceptions about feng shui. So now that you know what feng shui is not, it's time to discover what feng shui is—and how you can use it to change your life.

The Simple Answer

In the broadest sense, feng shui as a discipline is about the relationship between man and his environment. (Or let's be politically correct and say "woman and her environment.") It is about how energies react to those around us—both natural and man-made.

But feng shui is not a static art or mere philosophy. No, quite the contrary: It is as active and flowing as life itself. Because above all else, feng shui is about understanding, manipulating, and directing our energies to live, love, and work as wonderfully and productively as we can.

Thus, feng shui is not just theory. Rather, it is an intensely practical art, one that we use to change conditions in our physical environment to get the very most out of every aspect of our lives.

The Origins of Feng Shui

Perhaps nothing argues more compellingly for the substance and benefits of feng shui than this simple fact: Feng shui has been around almost as long as mankind itself.

Indeed, recent anthropological finds have shown that even prehistoric peoples used the principles of feng shui in an organic and evolving way. How? The way that primitive tribes chose cave dwellings indicates that they were very much in tune with how their "homes" were positioned toward or against the sun, in proximity of water, and hidden from enemy tribes. As civilization progressed, people all over the world began to see how their personal happiness, satisfaction—and often, even their safety—were the direct result of what could very well be called feng shui.

The Policy of Placement

Early cultures also understood, in a purely pragmatic way, how the placement of items in their immediate environments affected many aspects of their lives. For this reason, feng shui has often been called the art of placement.

Yes, early cultures recognized the importance of item placement, and this is certainly a vital part of the practice of feng shui. But it is very important to avoid the "quick fix" trap, or to think that putting a red ribbon in your hair will bring eternal life and a series of dates with Brad Pitt. (Besides, wouldn't it be boring if Feng Shui Chic meant always having to dress the same way?)

So here I tell you once again that placement is important—but placement evolves, just as life does. And even the cavemen, who changed residences with the seasons, knew that!

What Is the Meaning of Water and Wind?

In chapter one, we talked about the ideas of water and wind. Taken as separate entities, these elements have meaning all their own, because they are the forces of nature between which all other elements lie. But there is another meaning in which the sum is even greater than the parts of this basic equation of feng shui.

The combination of water and wind affects the climate, environment, and many aspects of our lives—including our chi, or energy. Yet this word, one of the most important in the entire language, has several other meanings. Among these is "breath." In all ways, chi is our own life's breath, an energy force from which all life radiates and grows.

What Is Chi—and What Has It to Do with Feng Shui Chic?

First, let's say it out loud: chee. (If you've been saying "chai," don't feel bad—most of us did at one point or another!)

Easy to say, harder to understand. *Chi* is one of those words that, like *shalom* in Hebrew, has many different meanings in modern English. It can mean energy, life force, or breath. It also means vapor, a nice metaphorical variation of its basic definition. That said, we instantly see why this concept is so very important to the study of feng shui.

But chi also has a larger meaning, one that is very much more than the sum of its parts. Chi is a "breath force" of energy—unseen but very much felt—that radiates life into and through all living things.

As such, chi is a focal point not only of feng shui and other Asian disciplines, but of Chinese medicine as well. Whereas Western doctors typically treat a symptom, Chinese doctors seek to cure or realign the body as a whole in order to have the body perform at its peak and to eliminate one or more medical issues at any given time.

Anyone who has had acupuncture or shiatsu massage already knows about chi. These practices are both based on the existence of a network of meridians running throughout the body—meridians that must flow unblocked if chi is to function maximally and we are to feel our best.

How Does Chi Work in My Environment?

Chi is both a pragmatic and a philosophical force. For this reason, it stands to reason that chi not only flows through all animals' bodies, but through all objects, even if they are ostensibly inanimate—or halfway around the world.

Interestingly, it wasn't until the mid 80s that we Westerners began to talk about the energy in a room, as if this were a nearly tangible force.

The energy of a space often reveals the purpose or intent of that space—the chi in a spa, for instance, will greatly differ from the chi in a boardroom, just as the chi of a 99-cent store will greatly differ from that of a couture showroom.

This is exactly what we mean by chi. It's not just an intellectual concept, but—and this is true whether we're talking about Chinese medicine or feng shui—chi is a very real, sensate force that we can actually feel. And now the good news: We don't need to passively suffer bad chi. By using the principles of Feng Shui Chic, we can manipulate chi to better our lives—today, tomorrow, and in all the days to come.

What elements affect chi? These include

- **colors,** which attract and nurture energy to create relaxation or activation. For example, a real estate agent wearing red might lose a sale by doing so. Why? Because red creates too much fire energy—and her clients, instead of signing the deal, could have an argument and storm off!
- **shapes,** which create patterns with forms. You can enhance energy by wearing flowers for a loving relationship, or to create flowering moments. These patterns are symbolic of nature and thus help enhance energy for the moment, and long-term, too.

- **lighting,** which can have great influence as well. The outfit you choose to wear when you command the spotlight—at a presentation or at your wedding, for instance—will differ from the one you choose to wear when you are sitting in the dark as part of a movie or theater audience.
- **temperature,** which can effect energy, too. What is the temperature when you enter a conference room for a business meeting? This can only result in "heated discussions"—pardon the pun—and non-movement of the proposals or ideas set forth. Instead, why not opt for a chill-out session—literally and figuratively.
- **scent,** something I probably don't need to tell you about; you know this one instinctively. What is your plan for the day? Are you wearing the right scent for work, passion, or power? Joy is no more the right scent for the office than a light, lemony scent would be for a night of dancing and romance.

Indeed, every element of our homes, offices, and other frequently visited places is influenced by the variables above. I will teach you how to achieve what you desire for every occasion by combining these according to Feng Shui Chic.

From the earliest known times of man to the present day, scores of people have benefited from the use of feng shui as it positively maniuplates chi. If you're like the growing number of North Americans who are already "in the know" when it comes to feng shui, you are benefiting, too.

How Does Chi Work on My Person?

While blood carries oxygen and nutrients, chi carries thoughts, ideas, emotions, and dreams. What you think—and the way that you think—have a great deal of influence on outcomes in our lives. This goes way beyond the rather hackneyed idea of the "power of positive thinking."

How is this so? Because chi is much more than a concept; it is actually an energy force that pervades both living things and inanimate objects. Thus (and this is a major raison d'être of this book), manipulating our chi has everything in the world to do with the success or failure, happiness or sadness, that we experience every single day of our lives.

What are the effects of disharmonized chi? Here are three prominent examples.

- Negative chi, caused by excessive light and artificial energy (such as air conditioning), can cause mental and physical exhaustion.
- Strong chi (like that produced by dampness and drafts) can result in two polarized attitudes, depending on the person: either excessive emotion and overexcitement, or depression and lack of direction.
- Fast-flowing chi (which you can feel on very windy days) can make one overtalkative and paranoid, fearful of personal attack.

Good Chi, Good Chic!

But what does chi have to do with Feng Shui Chic? Almost everything, as it turns out. Just as placement and position have everything to do with achieving the best flow of chi in our physical environments, so too does our physical countenance. How we dress and wear makeup, and even the food we eat, have a direct result on our chi.

And, why, precisely, is our chi so important? In Chinese medicine, it is the unencumbered flow of chi that is seen as a prerequisite to good health. Unlike Western medicine, which treats individual health symptoms, Eastern medicine treats the body as a whole. Thus, doing whatever necessary to unblock our chi is of prime concern to our physical and psychological health.

So, too, it goes with feng shui. Using color and placement to encourage optimal chi is what Feng Shui Chic is all about.

Need proof? Then consider the example of one of my clients, who made wonderful changes in her life by doing just that.

Sandra: Physician, Heal Thyself!

Sandra is a physician who received very little love and support during her childhood. Although she achieved academically, she was the product of an absent father and a narcissistic mother who felt her own needs were more important than Sandra's. As a result, she walked through her adult world with a profound sense of self-doubt—even though to other people she was a shining star. Indeed, Sandra, who was raised in the Mexican-American barrio of East Los Angeles, earned a medical degree from an Ivy League university and is one of the most esteemed specialists in her field in the United States.

During our first meeting, I noticed that Sandra was wearing black from head to toe. Now, this is not something that would have been unusual in the bohemian quarters of any large city in the 1980s; however, we were no longer in the eighties, and we met on a summer day when the temperature was well over 90 degrees!

Of course, my first question was this: "Sandra, why are you wearing black in July?"

"Oh, I always wear black," she said without thinking. "It's my favorite color."

Now, as a fashionista who lives in New York half the year, the attraction of black as a style statement did not escape me. But in the middle of July? And always? Something, clearly, was wrong.

It doesn't matter what your element is, or what season of the year you're in: Wearing one color all the time (black or otherwise) is not going to get you the happiness you want and deserve—in any area of your life. The feng shui color that brings you prosperity in one season is not the one that will achieve the same results in other seasons of the year.

With that knowledge, I diagrammed Sandra's feng shui color chart. We used both her month and element and her best color for season cycle to determine that she was a metal element. As we were in summer, I found her two best feng shui shades: khaki for day and burgundy for night.

Does this mean one has to wear all khaki or dress entirely in burgundy at that time of day, throughout that season? Certainly not.

What Sandra needed to do—just as you will—is to pick a zone (or life area) of most importance to you. These are the baguas I mentioned in chapter one and will discuss in full detail in the next chapter.

Although Sandra and I had just met, some things were clear. Her problem zones were not fame, creativity, career, knowledge, health, or power. Nor were love or support her primary problems, as she had a husband who (despite Sandra's deep-rooted psychological problems) had been with her for nearly fifteen years.

That left one bagua, and it's a vital one indeed: nurture. It was very clear from Sandra's story—even without the benefit of a psychology degree—that her problems derived from a loss of nurturing during her early years. Without correcting this problem, all her wealth and fame would continue to be for naught.

Examining the body bagua chart (see page 23), we saw that the nurture bagua is centered around the navel and extends to most of the lower stomach and abdomen area. In fact, when I showed my co-author, David, this chart, he nearly jumped up from his seat. "My God, Carole!" he shouted. "I think I finally understand why I've had stomach problems for my entire life!"

There is a simple yet very effective way to adjust the problems in this bagua: by wearing the feng shui colors that effect her best chi. And that is precisely what Sandra did.

From the time we met until our next meeting in the fall, Sandra wore clothing in the shade family prescribed by her nurture bagua chart. And when I saw her the second time, it was obvious that Sandra had become, in many ways, a new human being.

"I feel that life has opened up," she confided. "I no longer feel like I'm fighting everything and everyone, and that I'm more in sync with my own life."

Those words were music to my ears, and I think you'll know why. As I've already shown you, feng shui is all about putting oneself in harmony with nature, just as people in Asian cultures have been doing for countless thousands of years. By doing so, Sandra was doing exactly the same thing.

But Sandra had more to say. "I didn't stop with the nurture bagua, either. I had been having some problems at work, so I decided to wear the colors for my career bagua. I kept using the colors you prescribed for day and night, and—lo and behold—my career woes began to solve themselves. There really is something about this energy thing!"

Sandra's example is far from uncommon. Over the years, I have counseled many clients in the use of Feng Shui Chic as a means of adding power and passion to their lives. You will meet many of them very soon. But before you do, there are just a few more things you need to know . . .

The Body Bagua

What Is a Bagua?

According to Chinese philosophy, every situation and event in life falls into one of nine basic categories. Each of these areas is called a gua, or zone. It is a basic tenet of feng shui that these nine life circumstances are represented by divisions of an octagon-shaped chart, which is known as the bagua.

In the practice of feng shui—certainly, in its most common practice in this country—this octagon is configured or superimposed onto a two-dimensional "map" of one's home. Using this system, the garage might be the place for knowledge and your child's room the place for love. Under the rules of this program, you would adjust the chi in each room or part of a room (if the divisions of the octagon fall into two rooms) for optimal feng shui.

And what exactly are the life situations represented by the bagua chart? They are the following:

1. Career
2. Love
3. Creativity
4. Strategy
5. Knowledge
6. Health
7. Power
8. Fame
9. Nurture

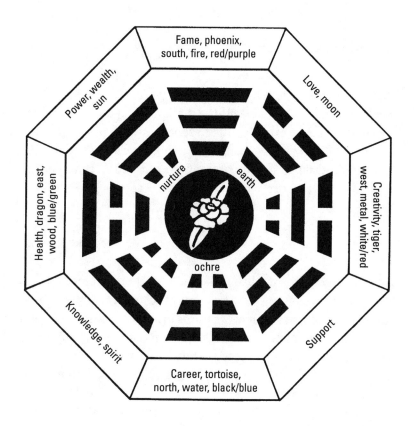

The diagram labels, reading around the octagon:

- Fame, phoenix, south, fire, red/purple
- Power, wealth, sun
- Love, moon
- Health, dragon, east, wood, blue/green
- Creativity, tiger, west, metal, white/red
- Knowledge, spirit
- Support
- Career, tortoise, north, water, black/blue

Center: nurture, earth, ochre

The Traditional Bagua

Another way feng shui experts use the bagua is by imposing the full map on an individual room. Frankly, in my experience, this makes far more sense, since trying to quadrant off rooms of a house (even on paper) is a tricky proposition at best.

Many feng shui practitioners take the bagua concept one step further. They use the octagonal chart as the basis of feng shui-ing a desk, car, or playing field.

How Does Feng Shui Affect Our Bodies—and Lives?

According to classic feng shui theory, we can achieve optimal health (or knowledge or wealth) by manipulating the color and/or placement of objects in that gua, or zone.

Doesn't it make sense, then, that we should be able to do exactly the same by aligning and harmonizing our bodies through the principles and practice of feng shui? This, in its essence, is Feng Shui Chic.

The Body Bagua

In typical feng shui, the bagua is used to align the home. In Feng Shui Chic, I have designed the bagua as a tool to show direction and intent—not of spaces, but of the forces in our own lives.

I created the body bagua to help people achieve balance between their minds and bodies—and to direct our intent within given life zones. By using the body bagua, you can understand how you look at the goals in your life, and then you can help stir the energy to help you attain these precise outcomes and aims. Call it a form of spiritual management—that's what I do!

On What Concept Is the Body Bagua Based?

Like all aspects of Chinese thought and science, the body bagua is an entirely organic system. In Chinese medicine, each body part has corresponding psychic functions, as in the following table.

Body Parts and Their Associations

Body parts	Emotion	Color	Zone	Season	Element
Bladder, kidney, ears, bones, head, hair	Fear	Black	Career	Winter	Water
Liver, gallbladder, eyes, nails	Anger	Green	Health	Spring	Wood
Heart, small intestine	Joy	Red	Fame	Summer	Fire
Stomach, mouth, lips	Worry	Yellow	Nurture	Summer	Earth
Lungs, skin	Sorrow	White	Creativity	Autumn	Metal

Thus, to maintain optimal chi, we must ensure optimal flow of this life force throughout the body. We do so by unblocking chi in each of the guas/zones (life areas). This is in all ways a two-tiered mind–body system that forms the very foundation of this book and the life-changing systems of Feng Shui Chic.

How Do I Use the Body Bagua?

Quite simply: The system of body bagua will allow you to be your best in all areas of life. By aligning your elements within a given season, you are "in the flow" and thus able to create harmony in your life. This allows you to make the most of your life in any given zone—and achieve the outcomes you desire.

You will learn to adjust your colors with the seasons when the energy is too high, and learn to restrain it when the energy is too low. By aligning your elements with the season, you can define and heal within a life zone. You are creating inner harmony to enhance your fashion style.

When you look at a map of the body bagua, you can see the

The Body Bagua | 25

process of real-life experience. You will also discover your style attitude in a pragmatic, yet beautiful, way.

The Body Bagua and Wellness

As you now know, the bagua deals with physical spaces, from our homes to our apartments to hotel rooms. And just as rooms have zones that relate to certain life situations or outcomes, so, too, does the body. It was the ancient Chinese Almanac that first correlated guas or zones to the human body, as long as six thousand years ago.

Which brings us to a very important point: The use of body baguas was the original practice of feng shui. Many Westerners have come to believe that spatial alignment is the founding force of feng shui, but this is patently not so. In Feng Shui Chic, we are returning to feng shui's very roots by using the mind-body connection to align ourselves and all of the areas of our life.

The bagua areas and their corresponding body parts are as follows:

Bagua area	Body part
Career	Mind
Love	Breast/heart
Creativity	Waist/arms
Strategy	Leg/foot
Knowledge	Hip/leg
Health	Breath
Power	Back/neck
Fame	Head
Nurture	Navel/solar plexus

Why Centering Yourself Works

According to Chinese medicine, your navel is known as your personal body compass." In Feng Shui Chic, you will learn how to control your emotions by adjusting your internal compass. Just like a ship's compass, your internal compass is a push/pull regulator, a tool that balances the self.

And how, precisely, do we center ourselves? By conscious thought processes and zangtra exercises, which will be part of every zone chapter in this book, beginning on page 80.

How Were the Body Zones Originally Derived?

Based on Chinese medicine, success in health—and life—was based on the unity of self with spatial alignment. It was the ancient Chinese *Book of Changes* that first correlated zones to the human body, five thousand years ago. This work noted that, because our environments are constantly changing, we must adjust (and align) our internal balance. We do this by constant adaptation, and that's another thing Feng Shui Chic will help you to do.

Please take a moment to consider the very title of *The Book of Changes*. I invite you to do so because this will allow you to understand on yet another level what *Feng Shui Chic* is all about.

In the West, we tend to think of finite, fixed solutions to our problems. Nothing could be further from the truth! Remember how I talked about "going with the flow"? This is important to do not once in a while, but on an everyday basis.

When we enter the zone chapters, the steps I ask you to perform allow you to clearly view your problems and issues—and, just as clearly, to envision solutions to each. You will do so not only by determining your best feng shui colors, patterns, and accessories for that zone, but by keeping mind journals, doing zangtra (a special breathing exercise based on principles of yoga and aesthetic medi-cine), and by opening yourself up to the visualization of your life's path—today and in the days to come.

At this point, you're just two short chapters away from learning how to make the most of each zone through the colors you wear on your body. But before you can learn to do this, you need to know just one more thing: your element type. Turn the page, and we'll do that right now.

The Five Elements of

Spirit and Style

At this point, we've looked at many of the concepts the Chinese use to explain the world—the very structure of feng shui itself. We've explored the notion of chi, or energy, and talked of the bagua, the octagon derived from the work of Confucius himself.

Now just one more system of thought remains between us and the practical uses of Feng Shui Chic: the five elements.

We know how important the environment and seasons are to all aspects of Chinese thought. And even Chinese medicine recognizes that the workings of our body are associated with seasonal cycles, such as birth, growth, ripening, harvest, and decay.

It only stands to reason that the five elements have such a primal place in Tao and other philosophies. According to Chinese theory, the entire cosmos is composed of various combinations of the five elements: water, wood, fire, earth, and metal. The five elements provide both a theoretical and pragmatic way of looking at the world's cycles. Yet these are not just symbols—they are real energy forces. Each element has its own energy flow, which contributes in all ways to the energy that all objects, people, and animals have in varying degrees.

How Do the Elements Contribute to Feng Shui Chic?

Both Eastern and Western psychology agree on one thing: We cannot change the essence of who we are. In the West, we talk of chromosomes and genes. Not surprisingly, Eastern psychology and philosophy focus on the flow of chi, as determined by our basic element type.

Can we change the very essence of who we are? Of course not. But what we *can* change—and this is the very heart of this book—are the outcomes in our lives. By using the principles of Feng Shui Chic, we can become as one with our environment, thus allowing us to make the most of the positive forces in the world at large.

Can I Be More Than One Element?

The first thing to realize is that none of us is exclusively a wood, water, or any other element type. This is so because the elements combine to form every plant, house, animal . . . and us! It is the interaction and interrelation of the five elements in each of us humans that informs who we are and how we act. It is the balance of elements within us that determines our internal climate.

That said, each of us can be said to have a primary element type, based on the month and year in which we were born. If you'll remember what I've said about the importance of season and flow, you'll immediately see that this makes all the sense in the world.

How Are the Elements Used?

The Taoist outlook is one of self-recognition. According to Tao, it is our job to not accept passively what life brings us, but to process life. By living in accord with nature, we understand our *own* nature, that of our fellow creatures, and of the Earth itself. Our element

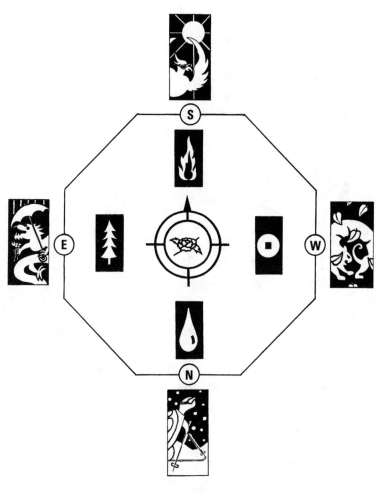

The Bagua and Its Associated Elements, Seasons, and Directions

The Five Elements of Spirit and Style | **31**

type allows us to know more about ourselves and about how our personalities and temperaments derive from the natural world.

Ancient Tao actually embraces five seasons of the year, rather than the four we in the West have come to accept. Thus the presence of the five elements, which coordinate to each of these times of the year in greater or lesser proportion.

The element relationships are as follows:

Water	Winter
Wood	Spring
Fire	Summer
Earth	Early autumn
Metal	Late autumn

How Do I Determine My Element Type?

The chart below allows you to determine your element by using the month and year in which you were born.

Element Type Chart

Your birth date	Element	Your birth date	Element
Feb. 18, 1912–Feb. 5, 1913	Water	Feb. 1, 1919–Feb. 19, 1920	Earth
Feb. 6, 1913–Jan. 25, 1914	Water	Feb. 20, 1920–Feb. 7, 1921	Metal
Jan. 26, 1914–Feb. 13, 1915	Wood	Feb. 8, 1921–Jan. 27, 1922	Metal
Feb. 14, 1915–Feb. 2, 1916	Wood	Feb. 28, 1922–Feb. 15, 1923	Water
Feb. 3, 1916–Jan. 22, 1917	Fire	Feb. 16, 1923–Feb. 4, 1924	Water
Jan. 23, 1917–Feb. 10, 1918	Fire	Feb. 5, 1924–Jan. 23, 1925	Wood
Feb. 11, 1918–Jan. 31, 1919	Earth	Jan. 24, 1925 – Feb. 12, 1926	Wood

continued on next page

Your birth date	Element	Your birth date	Element
Feb. 13, 1926–Feb. 1, 1927	Fire	Feb. 12, 1956–Jan. 30, 1957	Fire
Feb. 2, 1927–Jan. 22, 1928	Fire	Jan. 31, 1957–Feb. 17, 1958	Fire
Jan. 23, 1928–Feb. 9, 1929	Earth	Feb. 18, 1958–Feb. 7, 1959	Earth
Feb. 10, 1929–Jan. 29, 1930	Earth	Feb. 18, 1959–Jan. 27, 1960	Earth
Jan. 30, 1930–Feb. 16, 1931	Metal	Jan. 28, 1960–Feb. 14, 1961	Metal
Feb. 17, 1931–Feb. 5, 1932	Metal	Feb. 15, 1961–Feb. 4, 1962	Metal
Feb. 6, 1932–Jan. 25, 1933	Water	Feb. 5, 1962–Jan. 24, 1963	Water
Jan. 26, 1933–Feb. 13, 1934	Water	Jan. 25, 1963–Feb. 12, 1964	Water
Feb. 14, 1934–Feb. 3, 1935	Wood	Feb. 13, 1964–Feb. 1, 1965	Wood
Feb. 4, 1935–Jan. 23, 1936	Wood	Feb. 2, 1965–Jan. 20, 1966	Wood
Jan. 24, 1936–Feb. 10, 1937	Fire	Jan. 21, 1966–Feb. 8, 1967	Fire
Feb. 11, 1937–Jan. 30, 1938	Fire	Feb. 9, 1967–Jan. 29, 1968	Fire
Jan. 31, 1938–Feb. 18, 1939	Earth	Jan. 30, 1968–Feb. 16, 1969	Earth
Feb. 19, 1939–Feb. 7, 1940	Earth	Feb. 17, 1969–Feb. 5, 1970	Earth
Feb. 8, 1940–Jan. 26, 1941	Metal	Feb. 6, 1970–Jan. 26, 1971	Metal
Jan. 27, 1941–Feb. 14, 1942	Metal	Jan. 27, 1971–Feb. 14, 1972	Metal
Feb. 15, 1942–Feb. 4, 1943	Water	Feb. 15, 1972–Feb. 2, 1973	Water
Feb. 5, 1943–Jan. 24, 1944	Water	Feb. 3, 1973–Jan. 22, 1974	Water
Jan. 25, 1944–Feb. 12, 1945	Wood	Jan. 23, 1974–Feb. 10, 1975	Wood
Feb. 13, 1945–Feb. 1, 1946	Wood	Feb. 11, 1975–Jan. 30, 1976	Wood
Feb. 2, 1946–Jan. 21, 1947	Fire	Jan. 31, 1976–Feb. 17, 1977	Fire
Jan. 22, 1947–Feb. 9, 1948	Fire	Feb. 18, 1977–Feb. 6, 1978	Fire
Feb. 10, 1948–Jan. 28, 1949	Earth	Feb. 7, 1978–Jan. 27, 1979	Earth
Jan. 29, 1949–Feb. 16, 1950	Earth	Jan. 28, 1979–Feb. 15, 1980	Earth
Feb. 17, 1950–Feb. 5, 1951	Metal	Feb. 16, 1980–Feb. 4, 1981	Metal
Feb. 6, 1951–Jan. 26, 1952	Metal	Feb. 5, 1981–Jan. 24, 1982	Metal
Jan. 27, 1952–Feb. 13, 1953	Water	Jan. 25, 1982–Feb. 12, 1983	Water
Feb. 14, 1953–Feb. 2, 1954	Water	Feb. 13, 1983–Feb. 1, 1984	Water
Feb. 3, 1954–Jan. 23, 1955	Wood	Feb. 2, 1984–Feb. 19, 1985	Wood
Jan. 24, 1955–Feb. 11, 1956	Wood	Feb. 20, 1985–Feb. 8, 1986	Wood

continued on next page

The Five Elements of Spirit and Style | **33**

Your birth date	Element	Your birth date	Element
Feb. 9, 1986–Jan. 28, 1987	Fire	Feb. 7, 1997–Jan. 27, 1998	Fire
Jan. 29, 1987–Feb. 16, 1988	Fire	Jan. 28, 1998–Feb. 15, 1999	Earth
Feb. 17, 1988–Feb. 5, 1989	Earth	Feb. 16, 1999–Feb. 4, 2000	Earth
Feb. 6, 1989–Jan. 26, 1990	Earth	Feb. 5, 2000–Jan. 23, 2001	Metal
Jan. 27, 1990–Feb. 14, 1991	Metal	Jan. 24, 2001–Feb. 11, 2002	Metal
Feb. 15, 1991–Feb. 3, 1992	Metal	Feb. 12, 2002–Jan. 31, 2003	Water
Feb. 4, 1992–Jan. 22, 1993	Water	Feb. 1, 2003–Jan. 21, 2004	Water
Jan. 23, 1993–Feb. 9, 1994	Water	Jan. 22, 2004–Feb. 8, 2005	Wood
Feb. 10, 1994–Jan. 30, 1995	Wood	Feb. 9, 2005–Jan. 28, 2006	Wood
Jan. 31, 1995–Feb. 18, 1996	Wood	Jan. 29, 2006–Feb. 17, 2007	Fire
Feb. 19, 1996–Feb. 6, 1997	Fire	Feb. 18, 2007–Feb. 6, 2008	Fire

The Elements and Our Personality Types

Our element type helps define our personalities and predilections, our prides and prejudices. That's terrific to know, but wait—there's more good news. Your type also helps us determine your best

- colors
- fabrics
- patterns
- accessories
- scents
- metals
- dietary recommendations

Want to know more? Then, without further ado, here are the personality profiles of each element type, along with fashion and diet advice. But first . . .

A WORD ABOUT COLOR

You'll soon see the key colors for each element type. These are the shades that will stand you in good stead and will always provide you with optimal feng shui.

In the chapters to follow—the ones where we present the nine zones, or life areas—you'll find additional color recommendations. Why is this so? Because these are the shades you'll want to wear to achieve your specific goals, be they related to health, wealth, career, or love.

By combining your best element type shades with those designed to help you achieve your best in the nine life zones, you stand ready to realize your dearest desires in all aspects of your daily life.

The Water Type

An unerring intuition is the hallmark of the water-element type. To you, other people are as transparent as your element itself.

You can gaze into a mirror and seemingly make instant contact with the subconscious. In so doing, you can distinguish that which is true from that which is not. Artifice is your enemy, and you can discern it from a mile away.

Your true soul emanates deep from the interior; you give literal meaning to the phrase "still waters run deep." Of all the signs, you most need quiet time from the pace and pressures of the hurly-burly world outside.

But all this does not mean that you are reluctant to change. Indeed, just like water itself, you are the most changeable and malleable of the elements, both in terms of the practical and philosophical. Water elements have powerful transformations, moving as fast as the current at the mouth of the Nile.

Green is your very best color for periods of nurture. In times of

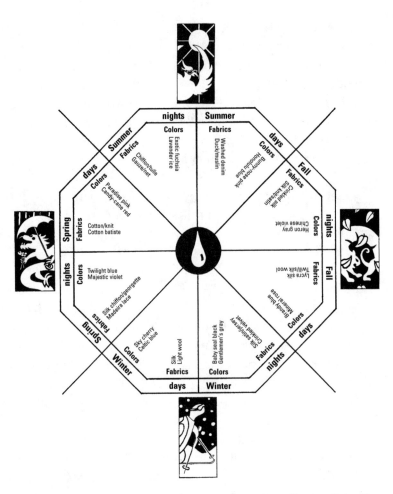

Water Element Color Chart

action, you will do well to use reds and plums in your dress, makeup, and accessories.

The downside? You can show all the cards in your hand, with too much emotion spilling out at inopportune times. This is because water is the sign of polarities. Day and night, positive and negative, joy and sorrow: You fluctuate between poles in a moment's time.

For you, there's no such thing as a continuum; all is either yes or no, black or white.

It's not surprising, then, that yours is the element aligned with indecision. You are an idealist who believes in "knights in shining armor," and the "pot of gold" at the end of the rainbow. You dream of hobnobbing with beautiful people and of owning costly possessions. Key advice: Never let these material things own you or dictate your direction and goals in life.

For you, every action has a concomitant reaction; there is no such thing as "letting go" or believing that things will work themselves out. This advice, then: Faith is the boat that will pull you to safety in muddy waters. Work hard during the day (rather than dreaming or putting emphasis on magical thinking), and let the stars work magic at night!

Sometimes, water-element people get all caught up in the whys and wherefores of cause and effect. When they do, they miss the action in the real world and the fusion of what really happens, as opposed to what they wish would happen. Don't waste time rationalizing. When you are finally offered the glass slipper, you can wear it, but until then you must concentrate on the here and now.

Interestingly, you are rather more grounded when it comes to other folks than when it's all about yourself. To wit: Community service is an important concern of yours. You feel strongly that all God's children have a basic right to food and shelter, and that you must do whatever possible to see that this is so.

This reflects on your highly traditional sense. You follow the mores and conventions of society, and you are in every way a good citizen. Similarly, you follow fashion trends rather than break them. I'm not suggesting that you become a criminal, but flying in the face of (at least) fashion might be a very good thing to try once in a while!

This is the sign of the overachiever who keeps fighting the battle until after it is won. As a water element, you need to learn to stop rowing against the current and glide like a swan. Go with the flow, and what you want can and will be yours.

YOUR STYLE PORTRAIT

Water personalities are the most fluid personas of all. Yet at the same time, there is a fundamental placidity and serenity to your nature.

As such, your clothes need to be nurturing, and they need to foster your calm nature. Calm, cool, and collected is your fundamental fashion stance.

SILHOUETTE

The circle is your governing shape, so think in terms of arcs and curves. Which means, lucky lady, that you get to wear body-conscious clothing with more panache than anyone else. As Belinda Carlisle sings in "Throw Me a Curve" on the too-hot Go-Go's reunion record, "But I'd rather be a pin-up girl than zero size." And so should you: whether you're reedy or Rubenesque. You go-go, girl!

COLORS

Pure, primary shades are what suit you best. Indigo blues, reds, and other clear colors are your calling cards. You'll always do your best when you choose
- Silver, for creative
- Gold, for power
- Black, for flow
- Gray, for initiative

FABRICS
- Stretch denim, for movement
- Silk, for flow
- French terry, to calm
- Linen, so you can breathe freely

PATTERNS
- Stripes, for flow and recognition
- Checks, for growth and communication
- Jacquard, for new opportunities
- Herringbone, for nurturing

ACCESSORIES
Stones do much to foster your relaxed nature. I recommend
- Pearls, for love
- Turquoise, for friendship
- Lapis lazuli, for protection
- Blue sapphire, for insight
- White opal, for vision

METALS
- Silver, for intuition
- Tin, for wisdom
- Pewter, for flexibility

SCENTS
- Magnolia, for beauty
- Lotus, for harmony
- Sage, for head-clearing
- Chamomile, for soothing
- Jasmine, for sweetness
- Myrrh, for reflection
- Patchouli, for flow
- Clary sage, for clarity

Vegetables	Beets, carrots, chives, cucumber, ginger, kidney beans, leeks, scallions, string beans
Fruits	Apricot, lotus, orange, tangerine
Proteins	Chicken, fish
Dairy	Eggs
Grains	Brown rice, pearl barley
Nuts	Pine
Seeds	Sesame seeds
Stocks	Chicken, miso, vegetable
Spices	Bay leaf, coriander, garlic, ginger
Oils	Safflower
Teas	Black, chamomile, green, lemon, orange

The Wood Type

The dawn, regeneration, and rebirth are all associated with the wood element. As such, it comes as absolutely no surprise that the season most associated with your element is spring.

Growth and expansion are your stock-in-trade; ascending to power is your driving force. You are the most forceful, stalwart, and determined of all the element types.

When wood types love, they do so with every ounce of their being. But beware: The unbridled passion you possess can ultimately be your undoing as well. The fire in your soul can burn brightly for the good of others, and many great social crusaders are of the wood type. Yet when left unchecked, your relentless nature can lead to wanton destruction. Of all the signs, you are the most fecund: fertile with the seeds of life and death, knowledge and intelligence.

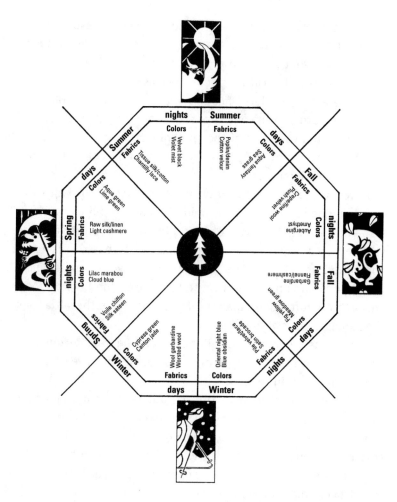

Wood Element Color Chart

Looking for a theme song? Look no further than Sarah McLachlan's moody tune, "Building a Mystery," whose lyrics describe a person living in a church, surrounded by voodoo dolls: "You come out at night/That's when the energy comes." Anything for a mysterious presence, that's you!

The Five Elements of Spirit and Style | 41

That said, you're hardly the shy, retiring type. Instead, you seek the limelight—though once there, you certainly don't give yourself away. In fact, your innate love of drama ensures that the performance lingers on long after the curtain falls.

A natural born leader? Of course you are! You attract followers by the strength of your convictions and your primal, even sensual energy . . . and your love of the spotlight promises followers galore. You are, in sum, the person everybody knows but whom nobody really understands.

Narcissicm, alas, is all too often associated with wood types. You have a tendency to place your own ideas above those of anyone else—and, in extreme cases, of falling in love with yourself. Yet, as with most narcissists, this syndrome may well be based in as much self-hatred as self-love. The prescription for your psychological health is to remain aware of these tendencies and keep them in check through frequent analysis of yourself and of the situations that color the days of your life.

New ideas are your most abundant and beloved currency. At times, you may spew like a volcano, and people will have no choice but to stand back in awe.

Your love of mystery can add drama and flair to your personality, but you should counter this love of the unknown by thrusting yourself into the sunlight. You are, after all, the element of rebirth! For this reason, you should enter the warmth of the sun and enjoy the colors of the rainbow, which will positively affect your actions and mood. Black and gray are the colors you should most assiduously avoid, because they have a tendency to thrust you back into the darkness, where you will wallow in your darkest, least attractive, and least healthy moods.

Wood-element people, as the very word implies, can be as strong as a sequoia—and as inflexible. You tend to live under constant duress, yet you must realize that much of this is of your own doing. Flexibility is what will keep you on an even keel and allow you to achieve your wildest dreams; remaining an unyielding tree will only stand in the way of all that you dare—and deserve—to have in your life.

Balance the yin and the yang in your everyday life. Enjoy the frivolity, drama, and oversized personality you were blessed with, yet come back to Earth occasionally, and the world will be your oyster!

YOUR STYLE PORTRAIT
At first glance, you're a no-nonsense dresser; froufrou and frills are not your signature style. That's because you let the sleek lines of your type hide the enigma within, letting the world know only what you want it to know. Building a mystery, indeed, you woodsy woman, you!

SILHOUETTE
A cylinder is the shape that rules your zone. Thus, a straight up-and-down look is the one that suits you best. Think of Faye Dunaway's classic sweater-and-slacks silhouette, or the straight, vertical lines she wore in *Bonnie and Clyde*—a look that's still a killer.

COLORS
- Peach, for health
- Green, for harmony
- Brown, for nurturing

FABRICS
- Chiffon, for health
- Satin, for allure
- Flannel, for warmth

PATTERNS
- Plaids, for longevity
- Jacquard, for elevated spirits

The Five Elements of Spirit and Style | **43**

ACCESSORIES
- Scarves, for energy
- Ribbons, for communication

METALS
- Brass, for success
- Bronze, for achievement
- Gold, for strength

SCENTS
- Bamboo, for flexibility
- Peony, for beauty
- Sandalwood, for sensuality
- Pine, for longevity
- Wisteria, for prosperity

DIET

Vegetables	Beets, black beans, carrots, cauliflower, celery, corn, eggplant, kidney, leeks, lettuce, peas, root vegetables, spinach, squash, turnips, watercress
Fruits	Black and red dates, figs, pineapple, plums, prunes, raisins, tangerines
Proteins	Lamb, suckling pig
Dairy	Eggs, milk
Grains	Barley sprouts, bran, brown rice
Nuts	Almond, lychee, pecan, walnut
Seeds	Sesame, sunflower
Stocks	Vegetable
Spices	Ginger
Oils	Olive, sesame, sunflower
Teas	Green, orange, tangerine

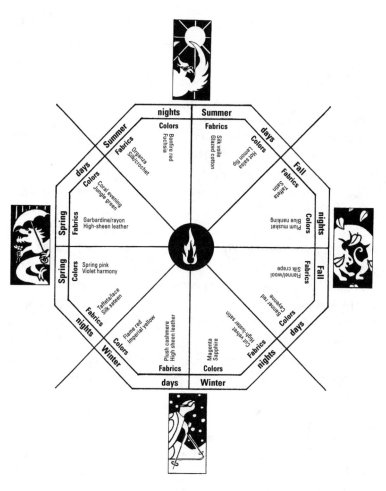

Fire Element Color Chart

The figure contains the following labeled text around an octagon:

- nights / Summer — Colors: Bonfire red, Fuchsia; Fabrics: Silk voile, Glazed cotton
- Summer / days — Colors: Hot salsa, Lemon flip; Fabrics: Silk/crochet, Organza
- Fall / days — Fabrics: Satin, Taffeta; Colors: Plum musket, Blue nanking
- Spring / Fabrics — Garbardine/rayon, High-sheen leather; Colors: Coral evening, Jungle green
- Spring / Colors — Spring pink, Violet harmony
- Fall / Colors — Flannel/wool, Silk crepe; Cayenne, Banner red
- Winter / nights — Flame red, Imperial yellow; Taffeta/lace, Silk sateen
- Winter / days — Plush cashmere, High sheen leather; Magenta, Sapphire
- nights — Cut velvet, High-luster satin

The Fire Type

If you are a fire element, you are a homebody above all else. But take note: Unlike many people in our sometimes too-glitzy society, I do not use this in any way as a disparaging term. Instead, you are a

The Five Elements of Spirit and Style | **45**

rock of strength and the anchor for everyone in your life. Fire elements are the first person friends and family call whenever there is a problem, and you are expected to offer solutions almost before the issue spills from someone else's mouth.

Yet you don't let your problem-solving prowess go to center stage. Instead, you maintain your power in the subtlest of ways, rather than giving the appearance of running the show. That said, you ingeniously let other folks know that your way isn't one way of doing things—it's the only way!

A flibbertigibbet? Not you. You labor patiently, even ploddingly, on projects over the long run, working assiduously where other folks would long ago have given up. Your organizational powers are second to none; once on a given path, you never waver. Others may look to the left and the right, but not you: You proceed in stalwart, straight-ahead fashion until you reach your chosen goal.

The downside? Fire signs, though often brilliant, can be inflexible. (Remember what I said about your way being the only way?) You stay with the tried and true when—at least sometimes—you should be exploring new, untested waters. "Hey there, Georgy Girl" (as the '60's song goes): Shed your dowdy feathers and fly . . . a little bit.

At times, though, your stubbornness serves a fine purpose: It slowly but surely brings others around to your way of thinking. You are a traditionalist who loves history—and, in fact, like making a little of your own.

You are magnificent teachers, leaders, writers, healers, and even CEOs. If you are a writer, you will definitely make your mark through the writings you produce. If you elect to pursue the noble teaching profession, you will shape the thinking of future generations. Your imprint is in all ways indelible.

Now, an apparent contradiction: You are loquacious when it comes to subjects of public record—science, history, and current events—but uncommunicative when it comes to your own life. So at once, you are a magpie and a clam. Your own feelings are kept locked deep inside yourself. Most of the time, you are a modern-day Mona Lisa; but watch out when your emotions do rise to the surface.

Only through balance will you achieve the happiness you deserve. Because you keep your feelings to yourself, you can become easily jealous, even touchy when you don't get your way. So widen your horizons and don't let momentary defeats get you down. Even you, wise fire element, can't always have your way.

If you think you're in a rut, you probably are. Jump out of that hole by trying new things, meeting new people, or by taking that Portuguese course you've been talking about for years.

YOUR STYLE PORTRAIT

You are known as the warrior of style. In fact, you inspire others with your unique and unparalleled fashion sense!

Your proud, undaunted—even fearless!—personality makes you hunt for exactly the right cut, color, and accessory. Of all the signs, you are the one who can find something fabulous in a vintage store and look like the belle of the ball. (This is especially fitting since fire is the sign of resurrection.) No one, dear fire woman, is more individualistic than you, and this shows in all aspects of your phenomenal fashion stance.

SILHOUETTE

The triangle is the shape that rules your element type. So make a beeline for an A-line skirt, dress, or coat. When it comes to slacks, be on the lookout for a gently flared pant to reflect the triangular shape so important to your feng shui type.

COLORS

Your best color choices are
- green, the refreshing, easy, color of nature that brings the seren-

The Five Elements of Spirit and Style | **47**

ity of gardens to our souls—and brings clarity to our hearts and minds

- blue, which represents harmony and peace and brings air energy to fire signs. Thus, royal blue is perfect for meetings and negotiations, as it calms emotions and inspires peace
- violet and red, which impart power with a vibrant "hear-me-now" voice

FABRICS

Think Cleopatra! There's nothing better for you than goddess fabrics like

- Velvet, for sensuality
- Damask, for prosperity, longevity
- Suede, for mental toughness
- Silk, for enchantment

PATTERNS

- Wood patterns, for enhanced energy
- Madras prints and checks, for warmth in the cold winter months
- Metallic threads, for success and good fortune

ACCESSORIES

- Metal accessories, to help balance raging fire energy
- One-of-a-kind or bohemian pieces, to fuel your creative side
- Scarves, for harmony—symbol of prosperity
- Beads and sparkles with which to lace your hair, to keep all eyes on you

METALS

- Gold, for power and achievement

SCENTS

- Neroli, for happiness
- Hibiscus, for splendor
- Gardenia, for sweetness
- Jasmine, for confidence
- Lemon, for cleansing

DIET

Vegetables	Artichokes, beets, black beans, bok choy, carrots, eggplant, potatoes, string beans
Fruits	Blueberries, grapes, oranges, papaya, pineapple, plums
Proteins	Chicken, fish
Dairy	Cheese, milk
Grains	Barley, black beans, oats
Nuts	Almonds
Seeds	Pumpkin, sesame
Stocks	Vegetable
Spices	Dill, parsley
Oils	Olive
Teas	Green, jasmine, peony, lemon

The Earth Type

As its name implies, this is the sign associated with Earth and all her bounty. If you are an earth type, you are concerned with abundance in all its forms. You love good food, big jewelry, and having more than enough of everything. *"Abbondanza!"* as Mama Celeste used to cry.

The Five Elements of Spirit and Style | **49**

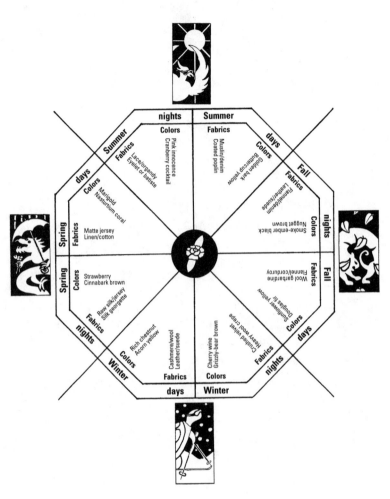

Earth Element Color Chart

But it's not all about having, as with water signs. Indeed, you love to share what you have with others. For this reason, you are especially good at service professions, in which you get to help and nurture other folks. You are a natural-born leader and would be perfect as the head of a small or self-owned business. As well, you might be very happy indeed working with a non-profit organization or charity, where you can show your love of humanity day in and day out.

Indeed, you are great at putting your own ideas into motion, but not at working cooperatively with others. As such, you shine as a salesman, architect, or landscaper.

Earth-element types are honest, efficient, and bold, yet you can be a very obstinate lady. You are as solid as a rock, and this can have positive and negative ramifications in your personal and professional lives. For this reason, the persona of the earth element is somewhat suspended in time and space, and even considered stagnant, as personalities go.

Yet despite your love for security and efficiency, you are also highly creative. How is this possible? Because you know how to harness your energy and use it wisely, rather than casting wildly about. You take calculated risks; yours is not a gambler mentality.

I'm sure you've heard of the phrase "one percent inspiration, ninety-nine percent perspiration." This applies more to earth-element types than any other type. You set a direction, then never venture from your path. When asked to do so, though, you can.

YOUR STYLE PORTRAIT

A slave to fashion? Not you, earth woman. If anything, it's the other way around: Your clothes have to work for *you*. Easygoing and straight-ahead, you like to look good, but not spend forever getting ready. That's because you're often more interested in the greater good than your own needs. Just remember: There's nothing wrong with taking a few minutes to be your most stylish self . . . then you can go out and *really* change the world!

SILHOUETTE

Square is your shape if earth is your type—but it's hardly your fashion forecast. In fact, nothing could be further from the truth. You'll look fab in a Jackie O, sixties-inspired silhouette—updated to the twenty-first century, of course. No flares or curves for you, earth lady: Square is hip when it comes to your type's straight-ahead silhouette.

COLORS
- Red, for an energy boost
- Purple, for devotion
- Orange, for health

FABRICS
- Satin, for power
- Metallic, for energy
- Brocade, to manifest your wishes

PATTERNS
- Pyramids, for power
- Animal prints, for intuitive knowledge
- Stars, so you can glitter

ACCESSORIES
- Triangles, for power
- Grapes, for a sweet life
- Butterflies, for high-flying happiness

METALS
- Copper, for healing and harmonious relationships
- Gold, so you can glitter in all areas of your life

SCENTS
- Bergamot, for clarity
- Narcissus, for flow
- Lime, for cleansing

- Lily, for nurturing
- Vanilla, for sweetness

DIET

Vegetables	Asparagus, beets, carrots, celery, eggplant, leeks, parsley, potatoes, radishes, spinach
Fruits	Apples, dates, grapes, muskmelon, orange, pineapple, tangerine
Proteins	Chicken, fish
Dairy	Egg whites, yogurt
Grains	Buckwheat, oats, pearl barley, white rice
Nuts	Almonds
Seeds	Sesame
Stocks	Chicken, vegetable
Spices	Bay leaf, garlic
Oils	Sesame
Teas	Peony, tangerine

The Metal Type

If you are a metal type, you are a gatherer; people flock naturally toward you. You love rituals, ceremonies, pomp and circumstance—anything that draws people together in groups.

Yet there's a great irony here: As much as you love activities that draw people together, you are never subject to groupthink. Of all the element types, you are the most prone to unconventional lifestyles. As well, you tend to have unusual interests in your personal and professional lives. For this reason, you are often miscon-

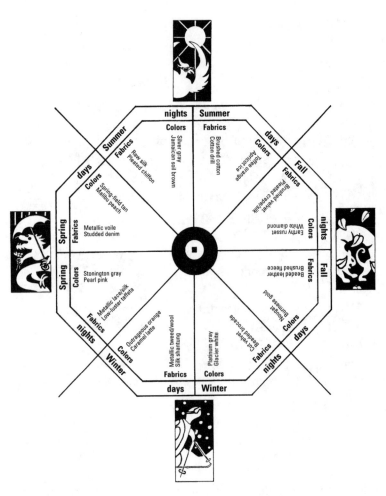

Metal Element Color Chart

strued as "bohemian," when in fact you are an explorer who loves all areas of life.

Physical exercise is very much your cup of tea. Why walk when you can run; why watch a game when you can participate in it?

Best of all, whether it's an active sport or board game, you are always the very best of sports. You are the sportswomen of the universe, and this allows you to adapt well to all of life's curves. Best of all, your good sportsmanship in all sectors of life is known and respected far and wide!

This stems from your basic integrity, which is second to none. Outwardly, your demeanor is sweet-tempered and even-keeled; yet you are a vociferous advocate of the abused and weak. Whether it is a family member, friend, or an entire group of people, you are an avatar of social justice in all its forms. From the micro to the macro level, fighting for what's right is a prime hallmark of your character type.

That said, you can sometimes mistake the tools you use—you metalworker, you!—with the outcome. You yourself are the element of change, not the tools or instruments you use in your personal and professional lives. Let light flow through you, and learn to accept the healing power of laughter. And do remember: The joy is in climbing the mountain, not reaching the top; learn to appreciate the view once you're there!

Of all the elements, you are typically the most artistic. More writers, painters, and musicians are metals than any other type. Beauty and grace are not only your vocational calling cards, but are the very words people use to describe you.

The downside? Your gregarious nature and wide-ranging interests tend to distract you from immediate and long-term goals.

In terms of relationships, you can often compromise too much—again, this is testament to your willingness to give in too easily. State your position and stay with it, especially when you know you're in the right.

The upside? Making others happy is your stock-in-trade. You are the supreme balancer of Earth and her gifts, and you want everyone else to share her glories, too.

YOUR STYLE PORTRAIT

You're high-energy, Miss Metal, so you need a wardrobe that lets you be as active as you are. Too-tight clothes don't let you breathe, and big, bouncy skirts won't let you move as fast as you like. For these reasons, the sleek and sharp look is as smooth as steel on you—just what you'd expect for the metal type.

SILHOUETTE

Sleek is where it's at for you metal types. Nothing flouncy or fluffy for you, nor is body-hugging your type. You're right in the middle, with clean, vertical lines, which perfectly complement your no-holds-barred, tell-it-like-it-is personality and polished poise.

COLORS
- White, for a lust for life
- Black, for creativity
- Orange, for desire

FABRICS
- Chiffon, for femininity
- Leather, for power
- Fur, to take life in stride

PATTERNS
- Animal prints, for growth
- Fruit, for fertility

ACCESSORIES
- Jade, for abundance
- Crystals, for clarity

METALS

- Iron, steel, and tin, for protection
- Pewter, for flexibility
- Coins, for protection

SCENTS

- Ginger, for the spice of life
- Rose, for wisdom
- Patchouli, for sensuality
- Peach, for a nurturing spirit
- Myrtle, for uplift

DIET

Vegetables	Asparagus, barley sprouts, beets, cauliflower, celery, scallions, turnips, yams
Fruits	Apricots, pears, plums
Proteins	Chicken, veal, venison
Dairy	Egg whites, yogurt
Grains	Bran, brown rice, white rice
Nuts	Almonds, peanuts
Seeds	Pumpkin
Stocks	Chicken
Spices	Bay leaf, garlic
Oils	Olive, peanut
Teas	Apricot, tangerine

Color and Feng Shui

In feng shui, colors are assigned metaphysical meanings that correlate to natural and spiritual elements. To achieve harmonic balance, tonality is key. In feng shui, color is never jarring or atonal, and no single color or color combination is used. The point/counterpoint of pale, muted shades and splashes of rich, vibrant strokes is always carefully considered—and this is as equally true of what we wear as how we decorate our homes.

The tenets of feng shui dictate that certain colors are associated with specific healing energies. In this book, you will learn to use specific energies to achieve optimal internal balance—the Chinese concept of chi—as well as to effect desired outcomes in your personal and professional lives.

Now, let's consider the basic properties of the major colors.

- **White,** which represents purity to Westerners, reflects mourning, death, and endings for the Chinese. Thus, white is used extremely judiciously and sparingly in feng shui—usually to enhance a natural background and blend with nature—and it is always offset with color (typically, the earth element, umber).

- **Black** is a water element that is sometimes used to balance other, less stable, colors. Black is said to "humidify" a space, infusing it with the virtues of water in a refreshing and cleansing way. However, an excess of black has a "flooding" effect that is overwhelming and can render its wearer dark and depressed.

- **Red** is a vital, energetic hue that invites happiness, power, authority, and fame. It is often used to remedy troubles as well as to capture dissipating energy and hold it in place. It is a provocative color that stimulates sexuality and romance. Red, along with its paler cousin, pink, can also provide love energy and cultivate marriages. However, given its potency and internal heat, too much red can incite conflict and stimulate tension, causing dissension and discord. Too much red can also cause burnout and has been known to create illness.

- **Orange** is a lively, happy color that promotes harmony and happiness. Of its cousins, terra cotta stimulates the appetite and peach can promote friendship, but also fickleness when used to excess.

- **Yellow** brings joy, good cheer, longevity, clear thinking, and tranquility. It also keeps us grounded, but we must be careful not to overdo the use of yellow for fear of turning an oasis into a desert with too much heat!
- **Green** is nature's favorite color. It reflects freshness, spring, and new beginnings; thus, it fosters growth, good health, prosperity, and fruitfulness. Green is often used to counteract and heal troubles of all kinds, and it is a wonderful antidote to poor health.
- **Blue** is the color of harmony and peace. It is a wonderful, soothing color, but must be balanced with earth tones to keep us grounded and focused. Blue promotes relaxation, tranquility, and spirituality; too much of it, though, can leave us feeling like our head is in the clouds!
- **Indigo,** the color of sea water, can be peaceful and inviting, and it is a sustaining source of food and nourishment. Like the sea, however, too much indigo may sap our energy if we are forced to struggle against its intrinsic power.
- **Violet** is a rich and vibrant color, the hue of royalty. Like indigo, violet is powerful, and when it is used in excess can be heavy and overpowering; for this reason, it is best balanced with plenty of white. As it pales to lilac, violet imparts dreamy, romantic moods.

The System of Feng Shui Chic

It would be easy enough to derive our program of feng shui style solely from the descriptions above. However, feng shui is based not only on color, but on direction and flow of the elements, and these, of course, change with the season. A certain color's effect is not stagnant; its power and meaning change as do the seasons of the year.

In addition, each of us is governed not by one static element, but by a yin-yang that is in a constantly changing delicate balance. This

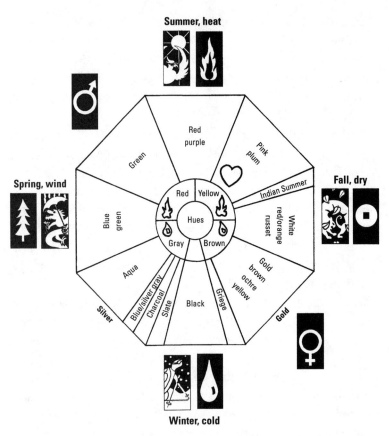

Color and Hue Chart

basic tenet of Chinese philosophy affects every element of our lives, from mood to health to economic success. Thus, in analyzing what colors best meet our needs at any given time, there is a yin (positive) and yang (negative) to keep in mind at all times.

This is all taken into consideration by the chart below, which is the basis for all areas of Feng Shui Chic. While the colorations will vary slightly based on clothing, accessories, and makeup—and have entirely different referents for scent—the principles on which these prescriptions are made are very much the same.

Your Personal Feng Shui Journey

Now you know what feng shui can do for you. Here, you'll find out exactly how.

Each of the chapters that follows is devoted to a specific life area, or zone. Once you have identified the zones that are most important to you, you will be able to use the steps in that chapter to help achieve your goals. From your personal financial statement to your dance card, you can and will attain your most heartfelt desires.

You may have thought, as did some of my private clients, that feng shui was about putting a red flag over your bed and enjoying a marvelous sex life for the rest of your life. It's not. And here's why: The physical part of feng shui, though the most obvious part of the process, is not the most important step. The mental part is, and as we learn to understand, we begin. By understanding that this is not a quick fix, but a process, you will understand the term "steps" as a process to move forward. Now, I'm not suggesting that you'll be old and gray before you see the life changes you seek. But I am simplifying this by asking you to understand and learn to first identify your desires and then take the steps—mindfully and physically—required to achieve your goals.

That's precisely why I like to use the term "steps," not "program" or "journey," but a process to move forward.

But I *am* asking you to understand that this is a function of understanding your desires, then taking the steps—psychic and material—necessary to achieve your goals.

As with many aspects of life, Tao describes the mind–body dichotomy through the classic concept of yin and yang. That is why this book—indeed, the very notion of Feng Shui Chic—is not just about outward appearance, but about our inner selves as well.

That said, making the most of Feng Shui Chic is an ongoing process of

1. determining your goals
2. focusing on your goals
3. achieving your goals

How the Journey Goes

It would be nice, wouldn't it, if we could snap our fingers and have our wildest dreams come to life? That's wishful thinking and not true to nature; happily, the program I present in this book is!

As we have already seen, the notion of applying the tenets of feng shui to fashion and personal style has been used for centuries in China and other parts of the East. More than a mere fashion statement, feng shui was used to signify class, power, the season, and/or one's mood. In addition, feng shui—applied in any of its forms—is about focus, intention, and flow.

Focus. Intent. Direction. These are what's key, and this is exactly what I'll teach you to do in the nine zone chapters that follow.

What are the identifying components of your personal feng shui plan? I identify them below.

THE KOAN

The koan is a Zen proverb, adage, story, or aphorism that has survived for thousands of years in China. These date as far back as Confucius. In fact, some koans were written by Confucius himself, though many more are anonymous.

In China, and in other parts of Asia, people have used koans as part of the spiritual nature of their daily life. What's marvelous about them is that, while a koan is sometimes metaphorical in nature, their pragmatic meaning always shines through. These koans are the ancient wisdom and explanations for the zones' purpose.

Here's one example: "All exist as a wonderful stream of life." (This is your koan for the career zone.)

Translation: With this koan, we see what we are where we are meant to be at any given time, and we see that our role is to nurture ourselves and those around us. In so doing, we solidify our place as part of our immediate environment and of the world at large. The koan is a wonderful reflection of the very basis of feng shui, which is alignment of ourselves as part of the world in which we live. (Indeed, feng shui is very much process, not the stagnant or static field that many Western practitioners—and books on the subject—would have you believe it to be.)

Unlike the zone om, the koan is not a chant, per se. Rather, it is an adage or saying, albeit one with highly practical implications. This koan, like all of the ones to follow, serves to illuminate and explain the basic theme of the zone in question.

THE ZONE OM

The zone om is an Americanization of the koan—an everyday translation, if you like.

You may choose to write your om on a piece of paper in lovely script, or in bold, block letters, and put it above your work station, next to your computer, on your bathroom mirror, or wherever you like.

How to make the most of your zone om? It's up to you—remember, this plan is all about choice. There are, of course, time-tested ways to best place your zone oms, and I'll share these in each chapter of this book. For now, here are some of my favorites.

- Make a printout of your zone om on a piece of yellow paper (yellow is a great career color) and keep it next to your computer, in your top drawer, or anywhere else where you'll see it often. Glance at your zone om whenever you feel the need, and get in the flow!
- Ask a calligrapher to make a small certificate to hang above your work area.
- Write your zone om on the back of a bookmark, so that you'll see it every time you open a book.
- Needlepoint your favorite zone om into a pillow or framable wall hanging. One of my clients, a sterling soul, needlepoints koans into small pillows and gives them as spirit-nourishers to those in need of a little sustenance. Now there's a friend we'd all like to have!
- My absolute favorite idea is to keep your needlepoint zone om pillow on your bed near you as you sleep each night. That way, the message can seep into your consciousness each and every night, and prepare you for success when you wake.

Better still is what one of my clients, Denise, did for several weeks. Instead of using her coffee break to primp and preen, she committed herself to spending a few minutes each morning to focus on her zone om.

Denise, thwarted in her present job, was focused on getting a new position. Meditating while thinking of her zone om allowed her to "be in the flow" (see below!) and make the most of her prospects.

On the way to the want ads, however, a funny thing happened: Denise, who had previously thought that there were no advancement possibilities where she was, was promoted within her department—to exactly the kind of job her boss had previously told her was out of her league.

Why did this happen? First and foremost, Denise opened herself up to the process. "It's funny," she laughed, "I'm Chinese American, and my grandmother, who's from Taipei, always used to try to get me interested in this kind of feng shui. I guess it took a little time for it all to sink in, and now I'm totally open to the idea." Because by meditating with her mind intent on her career zone om, Denise cleared her energy path and allowed three things to happen.

1. Her interest in her work increased.
2. Her level of professionalism heightened.
3. Perhaps most important of all, Denise became "in the flow," allowing good things to come her way.

With your respective zone—in the sector of career, love, or another zone of your choosing—you can, too.

An example of a zone om for career is: "The only way to grow is to be in the flow."

The Zone Profile

Here's where we will recap the very nature of the zone, be it career, nurture, or health. This will remind you of how this zone works with specific areas of your life as part of your body bagua, and how it relates to your personal feng shui.

You may notice that the order of zones in this book is somewhat different from that of other feng shui masters. The zone rotation I use is based on the teaching of my master, and it has a very definite rhyme and reason. By following the zones in the order in which they appear in chapters six through fourteen, you are inviting a constructive flow of energy—one that allows growth and new opportunities not only in that zone, but in all areas of your life. What's more, by following this order, you are taking your first step to becoming the master of your fate since you are taking a very active role in your spiritual and material growth.

Specifically, we go from the

- **career zone,** the embryonic state of our physical presence and form; to the
- **love zone,** where we manifest all our heart's desires; to the
- **creativity zone,** which relates to our development of soul and spirit's fancy; to the
- **strategy zone,** where we gain the support we need to do all things; to the
- **knowledge zone,** where we align mind and spirit; to the
- **health zone,** the area of physical presence and growth; to the
- **power zone,** where we shore up our personal influence and invite prosperity into our lives; to the
- **fame zone,** where we recognize our place in the world by learning both how others view us and—much more important—what we really want out of life; to the
- **nurture zone,** where we find our center and, by synergizing all the other zones, learn to love and trust our own place in the world.

Fashion Profile

Many women instinctively recognize that the color, fabric, and texture of their clothes inform the world of their focus and intention at any given time. These savvy women may not be able to articulate why they dress as they do, but there is an intuitive wisdom that works in their favor here.

And once you understand your feng shui colors and fabrics, you will have this same wisdom. Best of all is that this is a system you can use today, tomorrow, and forever. Compare that with the dictates of high fashion, which make sure that women spend money on each new style and trend. Rather than complicating your life,

Feng Shui Chic actually simplifies it, by allowing you to focus on your very best colors and nurturing fabrics above all else.

It is absolutely key for me to say that Feng Shui Chic is not about fashion, per se, and it is certainly not requisite that you be rich to reap its many rewards. And most important of all, Feng Shui Chic is not about blindly following fashion's dictates. In fact, quite the reverse is true: It is all about deciding how color, form, and texture best work to promote your own harmony—and in so doing, help you be at peace with the world.

Zangtra Mind Journal

As we've said before, focus, intention, and direction are the important themes here.

Many among you may already be journaling; congratulations if that's the case! However, this is a very specific kind of mind work that I ask you to do. Unlike free-form journal keeping, where you can write about whatever's on your mind, this is a very directed mind journal indeed.

As a first step, I invite you to light a candle as close to you as possible. You will find, I believe, that the flicker of the flame and the serenity and warmth that the candle brings will put you in the perfect frame of mind to reap the best benefits from your journal session.

Before performing your zangtra exercise (coming up next!), I suggest that you write down your feelings, emotions, goals, troubles, and dreams when it comes to the life area of note. Whether you choose to write in complete sentences, in bullet points, or something in between is your choice and yours alone. The format isn't important, either: You can write in a beautiful, bound diary, on a legal pad, or on anything else you like. What's important is that you do write down your thoughts and intents as a vital part of achieving balance in a given life area—and take the first step in making your wishes come true.

Please understand that there's no such thing as a right or wrong answer here. Do you know why? Because there's no such thing as a right or wrong life. Writing in your mind journal is all about exploring . . . about finding out what's right for you, not for your mother, father, wife, husband, best friend, or anyone else.

Of course, this doesn't mean that you should consider your mind journal trivial or fleeting. In fact, the exact opposite is true. A big reason why people don't follow their dreams is because they're not really sure what their dreams are. I see this in my clients all the time. By committing your ideas, feelings, thoughts, and dreams to paper, you are taking the first step to acknowledging them—and to following your heart's desires.

The list goes on from there. In your mind journal, do not try to ascribe blame, but rather focus on the root of the problem. By doing this, you will be one step closer to finding solutions to the problem at hand—and ensuring yourself that you do not repeat similar life patterns in the time to come.

THE ZANGTRA EXERCISE

The zangtra's ancient techniques are part of the heritage and hidden secrets that were given to me by my master. Zangtra is the name I have given to help this unique system of energy flow. This name is based on the system that stems from the aesthetic medicine, founded by the emperor Yan as early as A.D. 206. Zangtra is designed to be an integral part of how we align our mind, body, and spirit.

Zangtra theory is also mentioned in *The Book of Changes,* considered the source of natural science and the root of Traditional Chinese Medicine (TCM). *The Book of Changes* began in the warring state period of the Han dynasty. It later combined with the emporer's Canon of Medicine. Some scholars believe *The Book of Changes* is the joint work of Fu Xi, King Wen, Zougong, and Confucius. The book marries the schools of thought by Confucianism,

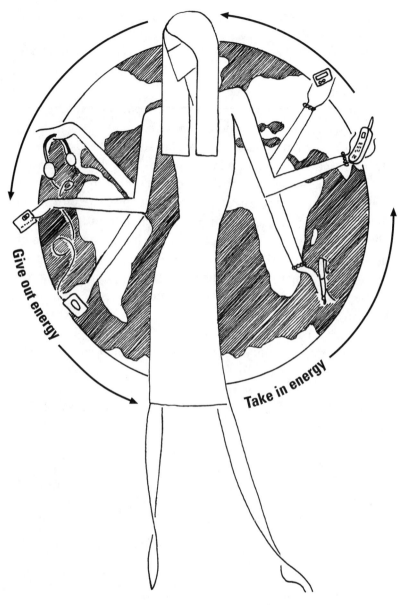

Give out energy

Take in energy

The Cycle of Giving and Receiving Energy

Taoism, and Mohism. *The Book of Changes* is the source of natural sciences and TCM.

By practicing these simple exercises, you will learn to embody the power of presence in the zone. It's all about action, movement, and change.

Through the ongoing use of zangtra body and breathing exercises, you will learn how to move forward.

Calm down! I'm not asking you to stand on your head or do anything of the sort. These are breathing exercises that you can do whether you're a marathon runner or in less-than-perfect shape. Best of all, you can do many of these routines anywhere: on a plane, on the subway, in a restaurant while waiting for a friend, or at home. (A few require a bit more space.) The choice is yours; many of my clients do these during times of stress at work or as time-outs during marital spats. It's not where you do zangtra, but how you do these meditation-based exercises that counts.

I am often asked when and how often to use the exercises. I always advise my clients that the best time is in a quiet place, day or night. A perfect time might be after writing in your mind journal to help you reinforce your thoughts, feelings, wishes, and desires. Remember, intent is everything, and by focusing on these issues while practicing zangtra, you are helping to visualize the reality of what you seek.

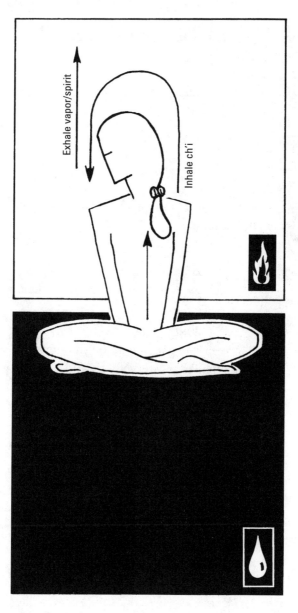

Exhale vapor/spirit

Inhale ch'i

Zangtra Breath

Your Personal Feng Shui Journey | **71**

Career: The Take

Ten Zone

KOAN
"All exist as a wonderful stream of life that is constantly moving."

ZONE OM
"The only way to grow is to be in the flow."

ZONE OM TIP
To keep yourself straight on your long and winding career road, paste your zone om above your car radio—and cruise into new opportunities!

COLORS | Indigo, black, gray
SILHOUETTE | Cruise into casual and go
with the flow!
BODY | Kidney and bones

Zone Wisdom

This chapter will teach you how to
- make the most of your current job
- learn to love work as part of your life--but not your whole life

- gravitate toward people who can help you in your profession
- steer yourself to a dazzling, fulfilling new career choice

Zone Profile

Many of us think that career success—whatever our field—is based on what we know, how conscientious we are, and how extensive our training is. Truth be told, these are just some of the factors that contribute to career success. Our personalities and predilections can be just as important as our training and education in determining how far we go in any job, or over any career trajectory.

At times, we all feel overwhelmed at our jobs. We can have too much on our plate, or too little—in which case, we fear that the ax will fall. If you freelance, it's either feast or famine—never, it seems, just the right amount of work.

Or perhaps your current situation is even more emotionally wrenching than that. Gone are the days when most people followed (or were forced into) one career. The good news is that we can have as many careers and follow as many interests as we like. But the other side of that coin is that there's precious little job security, and that carving our own career path is exponentially more stressful than the one-job days of yore.

Many of my clients suffer bona fide career angst. So if you're feeling downright overwhelmed about your professional trajectory, achieve balance through the fashions you wear. My advice: Large prints with leaves to alleviate stress and slacks worn with a red or yellow shirt will strengthen career opportunities for the corporate executive—not to mention her earnings.

That said, we can influence our success at work using the principles of Feng Shui Chic—and many of my clients have done just that. I invite you to start the steps of your career zone with your zone om. This will put you in a peaceful state of mind and will allow you to focus on achieving your goals in this zone.

That's just what Susan did. She was the prototypical New York career woman, and she had spent thousands of dollars on her trademark power suits. Trouble is, they brought her anything but!

There are several reasons for this. First and foremost is that Sue's fashion silhouette provided the very opposite energy of what she needed. Constricted from head to toe, she was more like a mummy than a maven. "Frankly, Carole," she told me, "I feel nearly nauseous every morning when I leave the house. I have a job that pays masses, has lots of responsibility, and even gives me the social position I always longed to have. So why do I hate it so much?"

I'm not a career counselor, but I do know my feng shui. So I replied: "Maybe it's not the job, Susan. Maybe it's the way you approach it that makes you feel ill at ease."

Peering through Susan's closet, I was regaled by her huge collection of expensive designer suits. Pretty, yes; expensive, definitely; but their body-binding silhouette was literally choking Susan and stifling both her career and her personal happiness.

What struck me next was the uniformity of color in her career collection—or, should I say, the lack thereof. Nearly everything Susan owned was black, a definite career zone "don't": Black drains you of energy and causes self-pity and emotional havoc, never good things in your career. How would *you* feel if you left the house every morning tightly coiled in black? This is exactly what Susan did, and a clear indication of why she was feeling so down on her lot in life.

I nearly commanded Sue to ditch the black and bring in the white, blue, and red that are the best hues for this zone . . . and to replace her tight suits with free, flowing forms like the ones I describe in the silhouette section a bit later in this chapter. Susan assured her intent by wearing the career zone accessories you'll also find here. After about a month, her attitude changed, her mind was freed up, and she is once again loving the job she worked so hard to achieve.

Black . . . and Beautiful!

Black, the favorite color of many fashionable women, can actually drain you of energy. This is certainly not an ideal situation, especially if you contend with the stresses and strains of city life. But if black's your bag, balance it with these energizing shades.

Color	Association
Red/Purple	Love, happiness, fame, power, wealth
Orange/Brick	Power, alignment with Earth
Yellow/Brown	Wisdom, warm and strong sun energy
Green/Blue	Growth, good health
Blue/Aqua	Good fortune, youth, smooth communication

As you'll recall from chapter three, each zone is associated with a certain area of the body—thus the notion of the body bagua. The career zone relates to your bones, kidney, and sense of hearing. Wearing white is especially important because it helps keep these organs in perfect working order.

The water element rules this zone. "Cruising" is your fashion outlook here. The metaphor is apt: Your goal should be to sail smoothly through all career matters—and, as well, through life.

Most of us find ourselves thwarted at work because we try too hard, rather than going with the flow. Now, of course I'm not suggesting that you can sit around doing nothing and all good things will come your way. (Would that life were that simple.) What I am saying is that a policy of acceptance and an agreement to go with the tide (not against it!) will put you in very good professional stead.

And please don't think that the water theme is merely a metaphor: Nautical motifs are welcome winners in this career zone. Personally, I think there's nothing so classic as a seafaring fashion motif, especially in the summer months. For some reason, whenever I think of that intelligent, inspiring beauty Lauren Hutton, I think of her in a sailor's cap and French seaman's top—it's a timeless look that is a hallmark of effortless style.

Boat patterns also work very well here, as does any theme with clouds, water, or sea. For women, a scarf or blouse is the perfect way to incorporate this pattern.

Fashion Profile

The koan and zone om for the career zone share a common theme, that of motion and flow . . . and so should your fashion silhouette. Think loose, flowing, and fabulous for ultimate career success.

By day, the best look for this zone is a loose cardigan or blousy jacket. This silhouette looks freshest when coupled with a black skirt, pinstripe silk shirt, or blouse adorned with water images or colors. Think Bali prints or clear colors and smooth silk textures— or, alternately, abstract and irregular soft patterns.

SILHOUETTE

Free-flowing, unconstricted garments work best in the career zone. Now, I'm not talking about togas and caftans; in any case, either would look pretty ridiculous in the business world. Instead, the silhouette here is as free as your range of career choices; just remember that constricted clothing is the very opposite of good feng shui. There may be a good reason the '80s were all about greed: The tight, power-wielding suits of that era were all about the wearer, leaving concern for others in the dust. Or think of how Julia Roberts got nowhere as Erin Brockovich until she toned down her skintight, breast-popping ensembles and opted for a (slightly!) more conservative look. I always advise comfortable, yet professional outfits that let you do your job while doing your best for others.

Feng Shui Do's

- Loose cardigans that let you move for comfort
- Capes and shawls with simple, elegant lines for adaptability
- Softly structured suits for success
- Irregular hemlines for evening for adventure and energy

Feng Shui Don'ts

- Any garment that constricts you: tube tops, super-straight skirts
- "Bondage" suits (think: anything worn on *Dynasty*)
- Caftans or djellabas: free-flowing doesn't mean huge!

COLORS

By peppering your wardrobe with more vibrant colors, you can enhance your career sector and bring more opportunities your way.

Feng Shui Do's

- Red, for health
- Gold, for good luck
- White, for kidney health and good chi
- Blue, to boost your energy at work and beyond

Feng Shui Don'ts

- Black, which can cause self-pity and negative emotions
- One red garment is fine, but too much red can cause mental anxiety and anger

FABRICS

In today's world, almost anything goes; but when the subject is your career, it shouldn't. Leave your leather at home (except for your purse, 'natch) and your Lycra for the disco balls. When it comes to career, natural is the niftiest choice.

Feng Shui Do's

- Silk, for a smooth road to success
- Cotton, for comfort
- Wool, for wonderful results whatever your career

Feng Shui Don'ts

- Parachute fabrics, which create an upwind and keep you fluttering through life
- Heavy wools or goat-hair blends, which portray you as bogged down and unyielding—a total taboo when looking for a new job!
- Nylon, which portrays you as flimsy and lackadaisical—a person who shirks responsibility
- Tussah silk, which is too thick and rough, keeping your emotions bound and you a tense Tessie

PATTERNS

Feng Shui Do's

- Bali prints, for exotic career moves
- Batik, for unconventional success
- Pinstripes, to show who's the boss—quietly and elegantly

Feng Shui Don'ts

- Triangle or flame patterns, which create steam—which, after all, is formed from water, and puts out new career opportunities
- Vertical stripes, which create confusing choices, not a definitive plan of action

ACCESSORIES

Feng Shui Do's

- Crystals and stones—clear quartz, crystals, lapis, and amethyst will strengthen your intuition and bring light and reflective elements to you.
- Dragons are the perfect way to bless you with great career energy. (Why do you think the Chinese so adore—indeed, mythologize—this creature?) If you're a nurturing, homebody type, turtles will do the same. Wear a whimsical scarf or brooch adorned with these luck-creating critters for career karma you'll love.
- Ribbons and headbands are surefire energy enhancers!
- Scarves worked for Audrey Hepburn and Jackie O, and they'll work for you.
- A large shoulder bag that is soft and pliable is both chic and practical—and, best of all, lets you go with the flow at all times.
- Umbrellas keep you out of the rain, and on a sure path to career success.

Feng Shui Don'ts

- Say bye-bye to biker chic (thank God, most of us already have). Car or bicycle motifs put you on a bumpy road, not as a confident woman sailing through a charted course of life.

Water energy is as changeable as a chameleon. It takes the shape of any vessel that contains it—and that includes the human body. The boundaries of a vessel—including the most important one of all, your own body—determine water energy's form. This makes perfect sense, since water is the most malleable chemical compound in the universe, as well as the most prolific and vital. Water adapts to space and form: as such, it deserves its reputation as "the fountain of life."

As part of the feng shui ritual, I'd like to recommend that you perform this zangtra exercise as close to a body of water as possible. If you're lucky enough to live by the ocean, nothing could be finer than going to the shore, where you can literally feel the bliss and bounty of the majestic sea waves. (And the seashore isn't only for summer; I personally love to feel a winter chill on my face as I stare into the great blue beyond.)

Not near the ocean? Then find your nearest babbling brook or gently pulsating pond. Unless you live in the desert, there's bound to be some body of water near your home. And if all else fails, you can do this zangtra breathing exercise with your feet dangling off the side of your local community pool. The scenic location is great, but in the end, it's the water that counts most.

Since adaptation is so very key to career success, it only stands to reason that the career zone is so closely related to the water element. I invite you to keep this in mind as you work on your mind journal.

Place a black candle nearby and recite or meditate upon this blessing:

Each force transforms into its polar opposite
Upon reaching its extreme state

Coming into being and passing away
In an endless cycle of change
I am part of this cycle
I welcome self
I am part of nature's cycle, to receive and manifest in life

After reciting or meditating on this blessing, I ask you to consider the following questions as you journal:

- First, focus on your intentions. As you focus on your career goals, breathe in the very essence of life itself. By combining water energy with fire energy, we receive the very breath of life.
- As you breathe in deeply, feel your emotions and write these down. These may include sadness, joy, fear, humility; feel acceptance and push through fear.
- Look at both sides of every question: The positive and negative poles are both important. Think especially of successes and failures in your career thus far—and remember that there are ups and downs in every career.
- Now that you are fully relaxed and at one with yourself and the universe, you may begin to record in your journal any associations that come to mind. Smell the four seasons; sense happiness; breathe in nature as grass, fruits, vegetables, rain, earth, snow, sun, ocean, and mountains.

One of the benefits of a career is that it shows us joy, light, and dark. Joy is for a few moments, with no worries. It provides us with the ability to travel beyond our immediate situation and to know that everything will eventually be fine—as it should be.

If we look hard enough, we can always feel joy in life, especially in our careers: the fast pace, the ups and downs, the here and there. It is your choice to make of this what you will.

In the end, remember: It is not just career success, per se, but the illumination of the self that is your best reward. The corner office and the house on the hill mean nothing without self-knowledge—and her sweet sister, self-love.

ZANGTRA EXERCISE

Your greatest reservoir of chi is in the navel area, which is the center of energy in your body. Chi always travels to and from this center, where all human attention and activity is centered. (You'll notice, as you become aware of your body, that when your breath is high in the chest, your chi goes there.)

The zangtra water position is immensely helpful in the career zone: Like gently rolling waves, it puts us in the flow at work (and in all aspects of our lives). To do this exercise, follow the steps below.

1. Lie flat on your back with your legs flat on the floor. Or you can put your feet on the floor and raise your knees, to allow your lower back to flatten to the floor. Feel the floor beneath you.

2. Place one hand on your lower abdomen and one hand on your chest wall.

3. Inhale deeply, allowing your belly to balloon out; notice that this action will raise the hand that you have resting on your belly.

4. Do this to the count of nine.

5. Place your hands on your sides and exhale.

6. Breathe in nine more times, through the abdomen, and without the use of your hands.

CHAPTER SEVEN

Love: The Queen

of Hearts

KOAN

"A huge tree grows from a tiny sprout."

ZONE OM

"The way to grow is to be less in control."

ZONE OM TIP

Place a calligraphied card with your zone om on your dressing table or bathroom mirror when getting ready for a date. You'll be telling the universe that you're looking forward to a great time—and maybe even a new relationship!

COLORS | Red, pink, fuchsia
SILHOUETTE | As bare as you dare
BODY | Heart, breast, shoulders

Zone Wisdom

In this chapter, you will learn how to
- open your heart to love
- nurture existing relationships
- find love in all aspects of life
- discover the romance you know you deserve

"Love will come knocking on your door when you least expect it." How many times have you given this advice to a lovelorn friend— or maybe even consoled yourself with this thought?

While there's a definite feel-good aspect to this modern-day adage, there's also a firm basis in feng shui for this point of view. Look no further than the zone om to understand why this is true: By letting go of control in our daily lives, we can begin to fill ourselves with passion, pleasure, and love . . . and begin to nurture ourselves. When we do this, we develop the self-love that allows others to love us in return. We learn to open and receive love—"Love grows" with time. We can't force it to happen.

Which leads me to another fascinating facet of this zone: It's not all about romantic love. Some feng shui writers and practitioners refer to this as the marriage zone, but by doing so, they miss the larger picture. Our koan says, "A huge tree grows from a tiny sprout." This tells us that by first learning to nurture ourselves, we nurture the world around us and all the people in it, and find the deeper love that all human beings need. Love of life!

Giving up control reminds us that feng shui is as much about giving up what is unnecessary in our lives as it is about amassing objects that can provide good feng shui. As you let go of the clutter and chaos of your past, you can begin to focus on your heart and all your present desires. After all, how can we find love if we're not living in the moment?

All this leads me to give some very ancient but very good advice: Put a song in your heart, sweetheart! Because if the mood music's there, I promise you someone else will hear it, too.

I'm perfectly serious about this. Living in the past will keep you there; but if you live in the moment, you're on track for running straight into love.

There's another very big reason why living in the moment makes sense: It's the only way to really know how we feel. "Get in touch with your feelings" has become a self-help battle cry, but there's truth to this call. I see folks everywhere—including my own daughters—fussing and fretting about relationships even before they've had a first date. Get real! How can we possibly know if we want someone to father our children before we've even laid eyes on him?

By the same token, a person is more than the sum total of their background, job, and geographic desirability, so stop placing STOP signs before you even hit the road. *Capisce?*

One last note on this subject: If people spent more time loving the one they are with rather than brooding over the one who got away or the one they *think* they want, we'd all be a lot further along the road to love. In the moment, baby, in the moment!

PREGNANCY

Remember that the love zone is governed by mother's love. This is perfectly symbolized by the unconditional love for our children, and helps explain why women are said to glow when carrying a child.

- From underwear to outerwear, it helps to bring in the vibrant sun energy. Thus, you can never wear enough yellow while pregnant. (If you grow tired of wearing yellow outfits, you can always don yellow undies or spice up your outfit with yellow hair ribbons, wrist bands, bracelets, or other accessories.)
- Pregnant women look marvelous in white satin semi-backless dresses. Bring more attention to your face with diamonds and pearls, faux or real. Or simply shorten your hemline and show some leg, keep the line simple and be beautiful. Wearing a racy red spices up a social outing, and is so hot that even the baby will rock!

Interestingly, the subtheme for this zone is mothering. The ancient practitioners of feng shui described a mother's love as the most selfless of all, calling it a "love treasure." In fact, they relate it to the unyielding abundance of nature—think here of fall's harvest or the overflowing water of a mountain spring. Is it any wonder we call her Mother Nature?

The zangtra elements of this zone are especially important because they will show you how to pave the way for love by

- destressing
- relaxing
- enjoying the natural rhythms of Earth
- seizing the moment
- relishing the intimacy we all seek

Decluttering our lives also lets us discover the truths of all our relationships—family, friends, and lovers alike. It also lets us understand our core values, which embrace our deepest emotional needs. Feng shui calls this our "inner knowledge," and it contains the emotional intelligence that is the very underpinning of all our kinds of love.

Traditional feng shui associates the love zone very closely with the number two. This is reflected most closely by the yin-yang (male-female) energy that underlies romantic relationships, but the symbolism goes much deeper than that. There is yin and yang—read this as give and take, up and down, more or less—in every relationship, romantic or otherwise. There are times when we must give, and others when it's our joy to receive. Flexibility is key, and the yin and yang can ebb and flow in a constant energy field. (The same holds true of same-sex romances as well as professional relationships and friendships.)

A gorgeous yin-yang with our life partners and friends is one of life's glories, to be sure. But remember again that this can only be achieved after we have discovered and cherished the joy of self-love and the treasures within our own hearts. That's the well from which all kinds of love spring. And do remember that nurturing our own self and spirit is not selfish; rather, it helps us create a warm spot within that unlocks our heart. When you have the courage to begin loving yourself, all other kinds of love will soon follow suit. That, more than anything, is the message of this zone.

Fashion Profile

In some zones, we dress demurely; in others, divinely. But in the love zone, all bets are off: I invite you to enter the zone of the vamp!

It's all about sensual energy here—and that doesn't come from traipsing around town like Marian the Librarian. Honey, this is the zone of exaggeration: the bigger, the bawdier, and the more bodacious—the better.

Good-bye, Georgy Girl; greet the goddess! Think opulence and extremes, and you're on the right track. Everyone loves to rib Ivana Trump, but the girl is laughing . . . all the way to the bank. And when a member of the British royal family first saw Elizabeth

THE BRIDAL PATH

What better place to talk about beautiful brides than in the love zone?

- Blushing brides white to cast a spell for marital harmony. When you become a vision of white, you're also using good feng shui to promote marital bliss.
- Best bet for bridesmaids: pink, another color that creates a lust for love. (And if a pastel-y pink isn't your bag, go for a modern hot pink or elegant dusty rose—whatever works best with your decor and bridesmaids' skin tones.)
- The marriage bouquet has its own Feng Shui Chic. Among the best blossoms to beckon bliss: orange, peony, lotus, hibiscus, plum, and (of course) rose.

Taylor's mammoth diamond ring, she cried, "Oh! How very vulgar." Yet Liz was never without a man in her bed, and the royals—well, you get the picture.

In the love zone, you're the glamour puss, too. Power and passion are your trademarks, allure your middle name. This, more than any other, is the zone of the female form, the one where you are woman in all her glory. Need a theme song? Call Shania Twain's "Man! I Feel Like a Woman!" your very own.

SILHOUETTE

Your sensual silhoutte is all about showing off your curves and of baring your skin—especially the shoulders and decolletage. Remember Jennifer Lopez's classic nearly nude Oscar gown? (How could we not: magazines will be reminding us of it years from now.) It's no wonder that she was wearing this so soon after her break up from Sean P. Diddy Combs. In essence, J.Lo was announcing her availability to the world about five minutes after she sent Mr. Combs his walking papers. Now, I'm not suggesting you prance around town in quite so risqué a manner—*that* might be dangerous!—but Jen was certainly on the right track by showing her sexiest siren self.

Feng Shui Do's

- A bustier, for passion
- A body-hugging jacket, for allure
- A voluminous flared skirt, to make an eye-catching entrance

Feng Shui Don'ts

- Structured suits, which keep you stiff and closed to love
- Tiered clothing, which causes ripples that may interfere with forging commitments

COLORS

You have one goal: to dazzle. So save the neutrals for another zone and get set to shine!

Feng Shui Do's

- Red, for power and passion
- Yellow, for relaxation and good cheer—a potent alternative to red, known as the fertility color in Asia (Note: red and yellow, not white, are the traditional marriage colors in the Orient.)
- Brown, for nourishment of self and those we love
- Pink, for love and affection (Little wonder we talk about being "in the pink" to denote our best and healthiest state.) And don't forget the kissing cousins of red and pink: from strawberry to fuchsia to plum, these are your passports to a rosy future.
- Orange, for dual appeal: This color is associated with both a stimulating, sensual love, and as one that promotes fine friendships.

Feng Shui Don'ts

- Blue, a cool color, creates chilly relationships
- Black, which denotes an emotional overload—never a good thing when you have a lust for love

FABRICS

Frilly and frolicking, sultry and sensual, leather to lace: These are the fabulous fabrics of the love zone. Smart and sensible? Not here, Vampy One; this is where you shake your booty and anything else you've got going on.

MENTIONING UNMENTIONABLES

Sporting underwear in a respective zone's hues always makes feng shui sense, but it's especially important in the love zone. Massage your body with color, and you attract the warm yang energy you seek. Sound strange? It isn't: In Eastern cultures underdressing (as I call it) has been a strong element of feng shui for centuries. Yes—Victoria's Secret can finally be revealed as a potent feng shui tool. (Tell that to yourself when you get your credit card bill!)

- Pink or red undergarments do the most to spice up your love energy.
- To balance this warm energy, green does the trick.
- A goddess bra makes a feng shui'd goddess out of you—and invites love into your life.

Feng Shui Do's

- Lycra, to stir up the fire in your lover (or prospective lover!)
- Leather, to show you're on the prowl
- Lace, to cast an alluring web
- Silk, to smooth the relationship you have
- Suede, to show you have a tough hide but a soft heart
- Taffeta, which creates the movement and helps rustle up love
- Cashmere and other soft wools, to make you warm and cuddle-worthy

Feng Shui Don'ts

- Canvas which is rigid
- Burlap which is restrictive
- Ramie linen . . . or any other rough-textured or unfinished fabrics, which invite tough relationships into your life—always a no-no, no?

PATTERNS
Love is in the air . . . with a little help from Feng Shui Chic! Put on these prints and start singing a song of love.

Feng Shui Do's

- Flowered patterns, which stimulate the senses and signal love
- Checks, which let you check out morning delights or love in the afternoon

Feng Shui Don'ts

- Irregular patterns, which show broken dreams
- Any abstract print, which confounds the senses and lashes out when love tries to enter your life

Diamonds: Forever Feng Shui Chic

The diamond represents new beginnings, union, and commitment. Be aware that its shape and color can affect the state of your union. Choose wisely!

Association	Stone's shape
Flexibility	Marquise, oval
Growth	Princess cut
Sensuality	Trillion, heart-shaped
Nurturing	Round, pear-shaped
Wisdom	Emerald cut
Harmony	Radiant cut
Association	**Setting**
Creativity	White gold
Strength	Yellow gold
Tradition	Rose gold

ACCESSORIES

You, a wallflower? I think not. Announce to the world that you're looking for love. You'll be ardent with the accessories listed here.

MONTHLY MAGIC FOR LOVE

The classic writings of feng shui tradition tell us that our best scents for scouting love are:

January	Orange blossoms
February	Plain blossoms
March	Butterfly, daffodils
April	Cherry blossoms
May	Wisteria
June	Hydrangeas, roses
July	Dragonfly, water lily
August	Grasses, morning glory
September	Chinese bellflower
October	Chrysanthemum
November	Maple leaf, peony
December	Peony

Feng Shui Do's

- Silk hair ribbons in red or pink are surefire love magnets.
- Metal accessories do much to attract love—wear them liberally and lovingly.
- Lizard, anyone? They're good love feng shui! So are alligators, fish, and tortoises.
- My own personal favorite: retro rain hats! They're best when matched with small handbags imported from India—a great fashion statement as well as fine feng shui.
- Love birds represent double happiness, and are perfect in a pin or pendant.
- Hearts attract love like nothing else.
- Red dragons give us the strength and power we need to best find love.
- An elephant with its trunk held toward the sky heralds fertility.
- The mystic knot is the perfect complement to a scarf or a shawl. (This is a traditional Chinese braided knot.)

Feng Shui Don'ts

- Jewelry with broken hearts and jagged edges which leads to heartache and unfulfilled relationships
- Accessories or jewelry with arrows piercing a heart which engender a rebellious and broken spirit

Zangtra Mind Journal and Ritual

According to Traditional Chinese Medicine (TCM)—the practice of mind, body, and spirit integration for physical and mental wellness—the heart corresponds to the fire element. It rules our innermost feelings. The heart also controls speech, and in some situations, our diets and emotions.

Mother Earth also teaches us that we must be part of a continual cycle of seeing, hearing, knowing, and doing. The following zangtra ritual and exercise will allow you to do just that.

Find a place to relax where you can sit undisturbed and in peace. This can either be a quiet corner in your home or in a serene place out of doors. Place a plum or pink lighted candle nearby, and recite or meditate upon this blessing:

> I stand with my body planted solidly upon the earth.
> The Spiritual Light of Heaven fills my heart and illuminates my Spirit.
> I light my candle and open my heart to give and receive life force Chi energy.
> I illuminate pathways to manifest passion for personal love,
> Passion for love of self, passion for friendship and passion for spiritual healing.
> I create abundance, harmony and Heaven on Earth.

After reciting or meditating on this blessing, I ask you to consider the following questions as you journal.

- What do I really mean when I say "I want love"? Is it really a romantic love you are seeking, or are you presently more concerned about finding new friends or resolving old issues with your siblings or parents?

- What love do I presently have in my life? Am I taking this for granted? (If so, you may want to thank the universe for your strong circle of friends and acquaintances, or even the love given you by a favorite pet.)

- How am I looking for the love I seek? The old song "Looking for Love in All the Wrong Places" hasn't entered our common consciousness for nothing; explore the ways you're seeking a mate or new friends. How might you change old habits for the better?

- How have I successfully attracted love in the past? How have I turned it away from my life? By examining former patterns of behavior—both successful and not—in your journal, you will start to see yourself more clearly. Remember, feng shui is all about clearing away clutter and making room for the new, and nowhere does that hold more true than in the love zone.

ZANGTRA EXERCISE

I strongly advise meditating three times a week before performing your love zone zangtra—or at least, as often as you can. This will reinforce the basic function of this exercise, which is to align your body, decrease stress, and allow your body to receive harmony. What's more, it will help you bring light within your body and form the perfect "O"—the smile that represents the light within the circle that you will learn to develop within your body.

This zangtra exercise helps you learn to visualize love and nurture. At the same time, it's a wonderful way to let out steam, reduce stress and anger, and cool your body from what may be an overabundance of yang (heat). To do this, do the following steps.

1. Sit in a comfortable chair with your feet on the ground and your back firmly against the back of the chair. Or, you can sit on the floor with your legs straight out in front of you, with a pillow to support your back.

2. Close your eyes and picture a red, circular stone. Now visualize its inner glow, letting it become larger and larger. Allow the warmth of the red to bring energy to your body.

3. Imagine the red stone in your mouth, and feel its warmth. Let it travel down your throat, to your chest.

4. Let this energy travel downward to your navel, which is your personal compass point.

5. Remember, as you massage your body with the stone's energy, to breathe in the fire and warmth, letting it relax and open up the flow of energy within you.

Creativity:

The Action Zone

KOAN
"First obtain skill; creativity comes later."

ZONE OM
"What is out is really in."

ZONE OM TIP
Place your zone om next to a bowl of differently colored candy in your family room or den to represent the wonderful creativity that beckons to us all. (I choose M&M's to represent the union of Meltzer and Meltzer; you can choose Gummi Bears, Jujyfruits, or any other candy you crave.)

COLORS | White, black
SILHOUETTE | Streamlined and cinched at
the waist
BODY | Waist, arms

Zone Wisdom

In this chapter, you will learn how to
- get in touch with your creative side
- find creative solutions to the issues in your life

- cherish the creative forces in the universe—and harness them to make your own life sweet

Zone Profile

Get rooted . . . get strong . . . and get ready to build yourself up, buttercup! Welcome to the action zone—the place where you *take action* to get your creative impulses flowing and growing like never before.

Why should you do this? Because contrary to popular opinion, creativity doesn't come to call if we don't. I know it's comforting to think that we can summon the creative genie—and genius—just by letting ourselves be open to both. But why wait for the muse to visit us when we can *be* the muse? That's what this chapter is all about. In fact, it's what this *book* is about: Using feng shui as an active force in every part of our lives—even our creative lives.

And that makes all the more sense since the creative zone is the action zone. Please allow me to say it one more time: Creativity is gained not through wishes and hopes, but through action.

So I ask you all to take one small but very beautiful step: *Participate in life.*

As style-setter Liza Minnelli asked in *Cabaret:* "What good is sitting alone in your room?" To which I answer: "What good, indeed?"

How should you participate in life? Go dancing, take up fencing, or learn yoga. If you're even more daring, then learn to rope climb or even mountain climb. All of these activities are great ways to let go, breathe, and become loose and relaxed. Just as top athletes understand the importance of stretching and strengthening their bodies to build power, so too can you invite creativity into your life by being loose, limber, and free.

Not the daredevil type? Fine. Participate in life by doing whatever calls out to you. A book club? Super. A cooking class? Divine. The act of participation and the joy it brings is what's key, not the precise activities you choose to do. (Of course, this said, I can't overstress the importance of physical activity; so if square dancing entices you more than rock climbing, listen to your heart and climb the career ladder with pride and joy.)

Why is action so key? Feng shui identifies this as the zone of the warrior—the one who carries the sword and is known as the "defender." This is the sword of wisdom, the blade that separates the roots from the seeds, the wheat from the chaff in our lives. Taking action also provides us with the inspiration to grow by learning something new—and it helps us to look within ourselves and, in so doing, obtain the inspiration we seek at any given time. That's what true creativity is all about.

The creative zone is where you indulge in your true artistic impulses. Keep your mind and eyes open to new shapes, concepts, and schools of thought. Take an extension course, attend museums, or take tae kwon do to get your creative juices flowing.

A fine feng shui tip: This is the zone of completion, so always finish what you start. Doing so allows us to create foundations for expression and action. When we become strong, vibrant, fit, and vigorous, we create healthy actions that let us direct our own lives—to be at the wheel, so to speak. Although some call this process centering, I like to think of this as "coring." It is the process that will give you the patience required to put down roots and a foundation on which to stand.

Before I go any further, a few more thoughts on the notion of creativity and why it should matter to you . . .

"But Carole," I hear you say, "I'm not really the creative type. What importance does this zone have for me?"

To which I respond: "All the importance in the world." Because the creative zone helps you achieve your goals and find satisfaction regardless of what you do, where you live, and who you are. After all, creativity is an essential ingredient in so many things we do.

Isn't it funny how we think dancers, artists, and writers are the only creative people in the world? I promise you that there are creative elements to every job in the world—and to every life, too. If you're an accountant (sometimes wrongly considered an uncreative post), you need to make numbers speak volumes—and at times, to present the numbers in a creative manner to achieve certain goals. If you're a warehouse worker, you will need to find creative solutions to changes in routing and products. And I hardly have to tell you how creative teachers—and stay-at-home moms—need to be!

Training our minds is also vital to the creative process. By learning to focus and by avoiding the delicious distractions that sidetrack us, we learn how to set the stage for creative riches. When you are in touch with yourself, you are building what Buddhists call mindfulness—the perfect marriage of mind and purpose. Just as the metal element in Earth gives our planet the vitamins neces-

MILESTONES OF LIFE

As you now know, this zone is marked by beginnings and endings. For this reason, I'd like to share a few more feng shui tips for important times in all our lives.

- When attending a funeral: Wear a green bracelet to keep loved ones in your thoughts. Wear this for forty-nine days, as this is the number associated with redemption.
- For christenings: Keep in mind that lucky charms inspire fortune. Choose a color that supports your child: pink for girls, blue for boys. Ask your guests to wear the appropriate color to show their support of the child. Give a locket with a photo of your child to the godparents and grandparents to link them as one. In China, christening bracelets are tiny padlocks that symbolize life and align the Chinese birth zodiac to the child by sealing your love.

Creativity: The Action Zone | 99

sary to nurture plants to grow, mindfulness connects you to your inner child.

This helps you draw from your past—it is the essence of "root chi." In so doing, we honor not only ourselves, but our heritage and those who have walked before us. (This notion, of respecting our ancestors, is at the very root of Confucian thought.) Undirected, unconnected actions—and, indeed, a rudderless life—are the very opposites of the focus we seek.

Creativity also comes from knowing ourselves. As a first step, I invite you to look honestly within yourself. Acknowledge your defects as well as your positive attributes. This will help you grow. Don't be afraid to ask others—friends, families, and professionals—to paint a picture as they see you, noting both the good and less flattering traits you possess. In so doing, you are entering a receptive mode—the true "zone" for creativity. The reward: a real vision of how you create and how you present yourself to the world. Learning to build upon your own natural resources is the "gold" that will let you treasure all that you have taken for granted in your life up to now. These are what I call your "golden nuggets," and they bring out your most creative abilities and visions.

Some people ask me: Can the image I present be multidimensional? My unwavering answer: Yes! You will find that your family shares one vision of who you are; your friends another; and your colleagues yet another still. Each area of your life is peppered with myriad abilities—some of which you may not yet have considered or known yourself.

Feng shui will teach you not to be something you are not. Just as a sheet of metal must not be too rigid, so too will you not be able to teach yourself to be something other than who you really are. Remember: To create suitable armor, you must be comfortable with the fit. The image of this zone is to develop it, fit into it, and use this armor. The chi energy of metal does not need to be replaced or hammered in. Let it work for you. Don't hide it—shine it. This is the spring from which all creativity flows.

To embody inspiration and create your centered heart, you must learn how to find the loyalty within—to root yourself and build up the power to defend yourself in the world. This act of expansion defines your body, linking it to your mental, physical, and spiritual selves. When you cut through the clutter of what separates your roots and your seeds, you start to develop self-mastery—your "sword of wisdom"—and find your truest creative self.

Pearls of Wisdom

Pearls, which contain the essence of moon energy, are representative of purity, feminine beauty—and creativity. Whether worn as rings, pendants, bracelets, or necklaces, from casual to formal occasions, pearls have feng shui meanings all their own.

Association	Pearl type	Color
Flow	Freshwater, lake Biwa	Gray-blue, black
Communication	Seed	Crème
Love	Baroque, mabe (blister), conch	Rose
Nurture	Natural, cultured Akoya	Golden
Structure	South sea	White, silver

The fall season, which governs this zone, teaches you to change. In autumn the leaves' vibrant colors reflect the change of season, and you can do the same—figuratively speaking, of course. Acknowledging and understanding your emotions help you get in touch with your true motives and allow you to move forward. (Remember, this is the action zone.)

What's more, connecting your desires to your spirit and inner child is a symbol of oneness—and of the female creative source that represents the moon wisdom for this zone. This is the zone of growing, learning, and developing—all forms of action as important as physical activity. Expand your capacity to love and to be loved by uncovering your heart's capacity for joy. Recognize your body's desires, take action, and you will always be in great creative shape!

And what about when you're not? What we call creative blocks are the direct results of inaction in your body and/or mind. When you are inactive, you move through life like a rusty saw. Action is the antidote here. To take positive action

- **don't stay mired in the past,** and know that sometimes we need to learn new skills before taking action. Our skills allow us to move; lack of skill limits us. The fear of being judged and of the unknown may leave you feeling insecure or not good enough. Identify, honor, and understand your feelings; use them as a springboard from which to leap to new heights. Remember: When you cut yourself off from your feelings, you can inadvertently cut off the creative process. Not only that, but by fortifying yourself in this way, you begin to transform yourself. The muscle of the mind is the thought and belief at the center of balance. This is the control dial that lets you create a positive path for your outer reality. Your dreams, thoughts, love, and respect always project energy outward by mindful action. In so doing, you are empowering yourself to an active, loving, and creative life.

- **don't be a physical or psychic pack rat!** Get rid of your baggage—psychological as well as material—and start to cut through the clutter to rediscover your most meaningful life goals. We can't be creative if we don't know what we're aiming for. To root, you must go deep to the core so that you can weed out all that—as U2 sings—"you can't leave behind." Chinese medicine treats the causes of illness, whereas American medicine treats symptoms.

Why not do both in your own life?

- **don't let rigidity rule your life!** This zone often shows resistance to fluctuating circumstances in our lives and in the external world. By looking for safety and control, we often sacrifice intimacy. When your soul stiffens, you suppress your extension, leaving no room for innovation and change. My client, Christa, is an ideal illustration of just this pratfall. Christa, a metal type, is an accountant. As hard as steel, she is all about control. The rigid application of pre-set systems are her very stock-in-trade. At work, she is a model employee, garnering respect from her boss and colleagues alike. Her home—even her children's lives—are run with the precision of a Swiss watch. In fact, she runs everyone's life *with* a Swiss watch. (Cartier, anyone?)

But there's a problem, and I bet you can already see what it is. By becoming so terribly rigid, so totally unyielding, Christa is interrupting the positive flow in chi in her work and family lives. And without getting too personal, I must also tell you that Christa's intimate life with her husband is as pre-programmed as everything else in her life—and this, as I'm sure you'll agree, is never a good idea.

By always looking for perfection and living according to a pre-

CREATIVE GEMS

You learned to love your element type's best gemstones in chapter four. But whatever your element, you can fire up creativity with the following sterling stones.

- Pearls, which illuminate all that you do
- Jade, which enhances abundance—in this case, of thought
- Citrine, to foster the sun energy that lets you accomplish all your creative goals
- Crystals, which impart clarity and vision

planned set of rules, Christa had created a tall ladder to climb—and a barrier to creativity and flow.

The first thing I did for Christa was to temporarily ban from her wardrobe the unadorned power suits she wore day in and day out. As well, I advised her of the importance of adding nine new pieces to her wardrobe, which is a key in this zone. That's because the number nine represents completion, as well as ambition and valor. So we went on a shopping spree and sought nine new items to spruce up her look, concentrating on a body-conscious, cinched-waist look. From form-fitting dresses to nipped-at-the-waist jacket and slacks outfits, we purchased only prime zone colors: white and black neutrals, with splashes of rust, orange, and red.

Just as these are nature's own harvest colors, so was Christa able to harvest the best of life in these dazzling new shades. And it goes without saying that we liberally accented her outfits with the accessories recommended on page 109. (We kept the clothing to nine pieces, but made an exception for the accessories so important to this creative zone.)

I also explained the concept of coring, which Christa agreed made great sense in her life. As well, I asked her to perform the zangtra exercise for this zone and to begin a mind journal, in which she diligently wrote for a few minutes every day.

The resounding result: a perfect fit! By adopting the Feng Shui Chic fashion advice and concentrating her mind with zangtra and a journal, Christa's former steeliness had melted. It was replaced with more caring for others and a newfound creative energy. "I'm never going to be living on a commune," laughed Christa, "but as accountants go, I'm pretty hang-loose. Best of all is that I'm not a taskmaster like before. Don't get me wrong—I take care of business," she continued. "But I also realize that business isn't all there is to life." I couldn't agree with Christa more!

And what would this zone be without family? It's interesting that we sometimes forget to find creative solutions for the issues related to those who are most important to us. But never take your family for granted. Honoring your loved ones is just as vital as nurturing yourself. By letting your family know how much you care and by creating honest resolutions to any problems you may have, you are also respecting your creative impulses in all that you do.

Creative "Tips" for Nails

The creativity zone is associated with the arms and, of course, hands. Keep your nails in tip-top shape to keep your creative juices flowing to your masterpiece, whether it be a watercolor painting, a gourmet meal, or a killer business proposal.

Association	Nail shape	Color	Accessories/ finish	Patterns
Creativity	Oval, arc	Blue, gray, lavender	Pearlized, opalescent	Moons, stripes
Abundance	Short, square	Rose, mauve, golden beige	High luster, airbrushed	Checks, florals, leaves
Love	Long, tapered	Bright red, orange, pink	Gems, rhinestone, glitter	Stars, zigzag, French nail with color tip
Nurture	Short, rounded	Sienna, yellow, browns, terra cotta	Matte	Natural, French
Protection	Long, square	White, rustic	High luster, studs, arcs, curves	Metallics, copper, silver, gold

Creativity: The Action Zone |

Just as coring is important in following your creative impulses, so too is coring your fashion mantra. Defining your goals is key—and so is defining your body. By cinching in at the waist, we make our creative successes . . . a cinch!

Body consciousness is what this zone's fashion profile is all about. Forget the image of flowing caftans and blousy hippie garb; there's nothing that calls out to creativity in those silhouettes. After all, this is the zone of action, so getting fit—psychologically and physically—is your calling card. Show it to the world with body-defining cuts and a cinched waist . . . and set your creative senses on fire! Think of how Janet (formerly "Miss Jackson") soared to fame after she lost mucho pounds and worked to achieve her present, sculpted look . . . or, the best example of all: How Madonna lost her baby fat, got abs and arms of steel, and came to rule the world!

SILHOUETTE

By belting our waists or tucking our blouse in, we define our body's shape. This is the perfect silhouette for this zone. By defining your body, you propel your entire being into action—just what is called for in this "action zone."

This is the zone of the classic and traditional. Surprised? Don't be. It's the clean silhouette and streamlined shape that beckons our creative side to sing. The alternative music maven Marilyn Manson once said (and I paraphrase) that true creativity can only happen in a repressive regime. This thought may help you better understand this apparently counterintuitive notion.

Think of jaunty Jodie Foster's classic silhouettes—or those made famous by Lauren Bacall. Neither lady is into flashy, in-your-face finery; both are famous for their tony, tailored styles.

Feng Shui Do's

- Jackets, for form and support
- Pleated skirts, which provide a feeling of regularity and structure—the firm foundation to being the most creative you

Feng Shui Don'ts

- Shifts or caftans, which are too formless and can't provide the foundation you need to be your most creative self
- Parkas and car coats, which are also too unstructured to provide the support you need for creative expansion
- Jumpers are out—you're a creative genius, not a bunny rabbit jumping from place to place

COLORS

In Chinese, this zone translates to the "white guardian." We Americans can identify this zone with the proverbial "knight in shining armor."

Feng Shui Do's

- White, to impart lust for life
- Red, to spark up desire
- Green, to improve your health
- Orange, to fire up your creative energy

Feng Shui Don'ts

- Black, which has a flooding effect and drowns creativity

FABRICS

The patterns of fall whisper of wind and echo the rustle of silk-like leaves. From cotton tees to basic camouflage pants, you can create your own special lineup in the creative zone.

Feng Shui Do's

- Cashmere provides the comfort and ease to be the most creative you.
- Velveteen knits to shantung silks are elegant, sophisticated, and oh-so-apt here.
- Chiffon inspires a feminine look.
- Fur-trimmed sweaters and jackets are the way to show your stride for that walk in the park.
- Leather can be your "sword," especially when you really need to make your fashion mark. I repeat: Who said tailored has to mean boring?
- Corduroy, for the grounding you need to be truly creative

Feng Shui Don'ts

- Vinyls and patent leathers are coated materials that don't let you breathe—a natural no-no in this artistic zone.
- Quilted or down fabrics protect you from your own creative impulses, as well as the world at large. To be at your most creative, you need to get in touch with yourself, not hide from who you are and what you feel.

PATTERNS

You might think that wild and crazy patterns rule in the creative zone. But ironically, the very opposite is true. Symmetrical, regular patterns like those listed below are the ones that let you be as creative as you need to be in every aspect of your life.

Feng Shui Do's

- Plaids, for the structure that lets you be your most creative self
- Argyle, which lets you blend into nature and feed your creative juices

Feng Shui Don'ts

- Tattersalls and checks make other folks want to cut you down to size, not acknowledge your creative abilities.
- Stripes present you as regimented, not someone who can express her creative side with a flourish. In this zone, you need to march to your own drummer, not follow somebody else's song.

ACCESSORIES

Learning how to accessorize teaches you to "mix with mobility" for any social scene. Since the tailored, sleek look is so key here, accessorizing for panache is what it's all about in the creative zone. Important feng shui tip: Wear five (bracelets, etc.) to represent the four principle compass points and their center.

Feng Shui Do's

- Silver fox, for love
- Panther, for nurture
- Tiger, for career growth
- Green tiger, for prosperity
- Black tiger, for travel
- Bird motifs, for good health and fortune
- Fish, for support and power
- Potted plants and tree motifs, for healing and growth
- White cranes, to strengthen all your relationships

- Lockets and charms with photographs, to strengthen family ties and inspiring relationships
- Seascapes and waves, to promote support in all life areas
- Fruit, which promotes strong health and peaceful family relationships

Feng Shui Don'ts

- Knotted ropes and safety pins, which show you need mending
- Rough edges on pins or brooches, which don't let your creativity flow as it should
- Guns, as they show you're ready to fight, not to fill the world with creative love

Zangtra Mind Journal and Ritual

Light a green candle for growth or a harvest orange one for nurturing. Take in a breath, then enjoy the candles' scent. Realize that by taking a break, you allow the way for mental expansion. Use this blessing for your meditation times:

> *As I light this flame*
> *I begin my meditation*
> *Listening for the Ancient whispers*
> *Of Ancestral wisdom.*
> *"A great fire may follow a single spark,"*
> *Says one of the ancient Koans.*
> *I meditate on the riddle*
> *And seek enlightenment;*
> *A single intuitive spark*
> *Fuels the fire of understanding.*
> *I give thanks for the abundance of life*
> *And welcome harmony, prosperity and love.*

You are in the zone of endings and beginnings. This "prime time" zone looks both forward and back, and by looking to the future you can put your life in place. The primary metal is gold. For this reason, think of your golden years and of what you want to be like then. Then design a program that lets you become that person.

Have an idea, a beginning, a starting point. Structure and strategize your thoughts into an outline. I like to categorize my thoughts like this.

A. Feelings: Begin a journal of your feelings and emotions.
B. Acceptance: Ask yourself what your fears are, what makes you sad, and what brings you joy.
C. Goals: Visualize your goals. Set simple goals, structure them in a simple way, and achieve them by simplifying.
D. Outcome: Harnessing power allows you to create in tangible form and provides movement from raw ideas to focused energy. (Remember: Everything you create is a movement. As you move in a full circle, you spiral from one event to the next.)
E. Balance: More than anything, balance provides confidence, which is based on purity. Center yourself; accept your own strengths and limits.
F. Joy: Remember that all joy bears truth at the root. Enjoy what you are doing and know that joy will come!

Now, be very specific. Ask yourself:

- What are my major creative goals?
- How can I foster my creative impulses?
- What do I mean by "creativity," and why do I need this in my life?
- What activities help me be my most creative self?

ZANGTRA EXERCISE

By visualizing your body's structure and form you will connect to your bone structure. This is your house of support. This exercise is necessary to help you create a strong back, offering protection and back support. Feng shui tip: Think of yourself as a plant in the

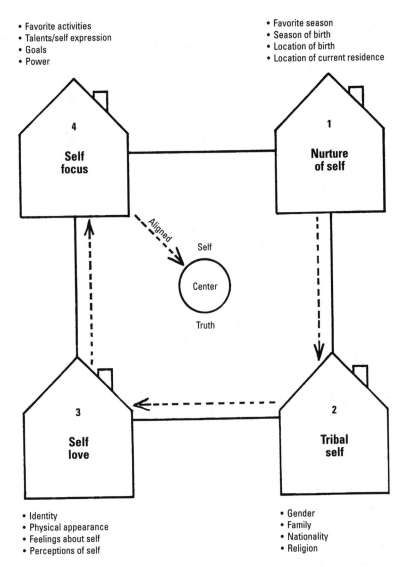

- Favorite activities
- Talents/self expression
- Goals
- Power

- Favorite season
- Season of birth
- Location of birth
- Location of current residence

4

Self focus

1

Nurture of self

Aligned

Self

Center

Truth

3

Self love

2

Tribal self

- Identity
- Physical appearance
- Feelings about self
- Perceptions of self

- Gender
- Family
- Nationality
- Religion

Zangtra Support

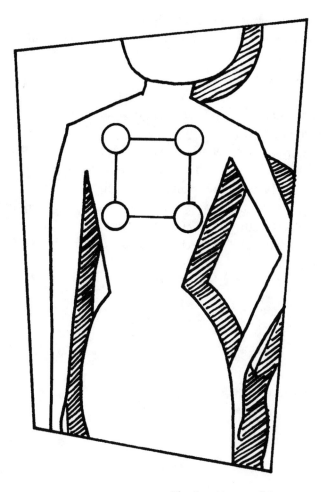

The Four Houses of Support

ground. Learn to become one with the earth, nurturing and rooting yourself.

To perform this exercise follow these steps:

1. Stand straight with your feet approximately three to six inches apart.

2. Do not lean front or back or side to side.
3. Drop your head forward and release the tension in your neck. Let go, and by letting go your muscles will relax, bringing your shoulders downward.
4. To create back support, visualize your spinal structure as a pagoda supporting upward from your sacrum; this is chi energy building upward.
5. Now bring this chi energy downward to behind your knees. Feel the energy traveling to your heels, and as the chi energy connects, feel your feet connect to the earth.
6. Gently press down on your back for support, thus aligning the skeletal structure. Press and release three times. Feel the chi energy flowing and connecting your back with your legs to your feet.

Strategy:

The Support Zone

KOAN
"By seeking something new, you arrive at the understanding of an ancient thing."

ZONE OM
"Open your spirit to light and love."

ZONE OM TIP
Stick a Post-it with your zone om next to your computer . . . and all the information coming in will support your fondest hopes and dreams.

COLORS | Yellow, orange
SILHOUETTE | Sleek, elongated
BODY | Hip, leg, foot

Zone Wisdom

In this chapter, you will learn how to
- understand the power of strategic thinking
- find strategic solutions to specific issues in your personal and professional lives
- use strategic skills to get all that you want out of life

Zone Profile

Strategy. It's a word we hear a lot of these days—especially if we have an MBA in the family. But believe me, you don't have to be an advertising executive or Donald Trump to know that strategy is an important part of our daily lives.

So what, then, does strategy really mean? My dictionary describes it as the science or art of planning or directing. Now, you tell me: Is that something only an MBA needs to know about? I think not.

In other words, all of us need to use a little strategy every day of the year. Or, as one of my friends is always telling her hedonistic daughter: "Honey, think about where you want to land before jumping off the bridge!"

I know, I know—our lives are busier today than we ever could have dreamed possible. Finding five minutes for ourselves is no mean feat, let alone the time required to strategize. Yet strategize we must if we are to make the most of our lives, instead of running pell-mell from one project . . . one job . . . or one lover to the next. Suffice it to say that this is a hugely important zone.

Boiled down to the essence, your mantra for this zone is this: "Create wisdom for strategic success." In this zone, you'll learn to clear the way for strategic vision in order to do just that.

Interestingly, the teachings of feng shui identify the strategy zone with fatherhood. This zone represents male energy, along with financial abundance. What's more, the strategy zone is closely associated with leadership and your ability to "step up to the plate." As you know from the previous chapter, sports metaphors often reflect the rules of life—and nowhere is this more apparent than in the strategy zone.

Most of us think of strategy as some kind of grand plan, with a dizzy parade of facts and figures. Not so! In fact, according to Chinese thought, wisdom comes not from amassing new bodies of information, but from letting go of old ways of thinking. How is this possible? Because when we clear out the cobwebs from our mind, we create openness for expansion—of knowledge and power. By organizing existing information and thoughtforms, we can restore balance. In so doing, we simplify our lives and provide ourselves with a clear new vision of who we are, where we are, and what we seek to do.

The most beautiful part of this simplification process is that it allows us to gain both physical and psychological support from our newly balanced chi. And if you'll recall, chi means not only spirit, but breath—so the zangtra breathing exercises that follow are especially important in this zone.

For now, know this: By learning to develop your chi/breath, you are taking a first giant step to turning your dreams into reality. In developing your breath support, you are learning to embody your physical self. This is so because chi, literally and figuratively, is the very center of your body support, providing as it does the very breath of life. As I tell my clients nearly every day: "Your breath can set you free."

There's another wonderful result of getting your chi in tip-top shape: It aligns you not only within yourself, but to the world as a whole. Remember what we said earlier about feng shui stemming from the natural world? Healthy chi means a firm base of support, your rooting to the world, and that helps us achieve strong relationships with the rest of the world.

Letting your chi flow at its smoothest also creates an uncluttered self that provides a strong foundation for all aspects of your life. When we do this, we achieve the advice of our zone om: We open our spirit to light and love. Good chi provides us with the energy to move mountains—or at least turn a few of those mountains into molehills!

First I'd like to share a story with you. It's about my client, Kevin, a golf pro at a well-known resort. For no apparent reason, Kevin started having trouble with his game. It seemed that the more effort he exerted in correcting his swing, the worse things became. His whole body tightened up and his breath constricted. Not only did this block the flow of his chi energy, but it fouled up the natural rhythm of his formerly suave swing.

Things got even worse. The more Kevin concentrated on correcting his posture and swing, the less he was able to focus on the strategy of his game. Just like Kevin Costner in *Tin Cup,* he needed to unblock his fear of failure in order to empower himself to gain a firm footing for success. (See how the foot is the perfect physical and figurative image for this zone?)

Support Hose

The legs and feet are associated with the strategy zone, and for good reason—before you reach for the stars, it helps to first have your feet planted firmly on the ground. Of course, the first step in any journey is to put one well-shod foot in front of the other, but don't forget your support hose. Choose the color and/or pattern to attract the energy you need to realize *your* dreams.

Association	Color	Pattern
Flexibility	Blue, black, gray	Waves, nautical, washed heather
Prosperity	Blue, green, red	Checks, argyle, logos
Love	Red, purple, pink, plum	Stars, triangles, herringbone, flowers
Nurture	Yellow, brown, natural	Tweeds, leaves, plaids, botanical
Structure	White, orange, metallic	Houndstooth, animal motif, stripes

To succeed at golf—or at anything in life—you need to be fully focused and free of clutter in the area directly above your shoulders. (Yes, I'm talking about your noggin.) In a phrase, you need to be fully present and in the moment. You must align your mind and body with the action at hand, be it a game of golf, a project at work, or setting your sights on a new object of love.

Indeed, for Kevin, hitting the ball with a seven iron is no different from the samurai of yore using his sword and blade in battle. Both require complete focus and a steadfast plan of action. Patience and concentration are your swords. Use them well, and your destiny is in the palm of your hands.

By restoring his chi to perfect balance by wearing the right colors and performing zangtra exercise, Kevin was able to quickly return to his erstwhile, winning form. I've said it before, but I'll say it again: With balanced chi, we have renewed energy; by letting go and being in the flow, we free our bodies and minds to achieve whatever it is that we want.

Just like Kevin did, we can use our breath to relax and center our entire beings. In this way, we can all create our very personal holes in one.

One last thought. By clearing the clutter from our minds, we clear it from our hearts as well. This lets us open up our senses, open our hearts, and open delicious new doors. As our koan informs us, this also allows us to arrive at an understanding of old issues in our lives. Think of this as a mental vacation, and allow yourself to reap all the bounties of your trip (even if it's just to a nearby park to smell the new spring flowers).

Getting back to basics—and following the Feng Shui Chic advice here—lets you marry a new wardrobe with an uncluttered, fresh mind. With an open heart and mind, who knows what you'll discover—or whom you'll meet? Be kind to your soul, experience all the possibilities, and follow your heart's desires.

Given this example, is it any surprise, then, that the body parts

TRAVEL TIPS

While the main focus of this life area is on support, this is also the zone that governs travel. It makes perfect sense, because you now know that by finding our footing—firm support—we're able to expand. And what could be more expansive for our minds and souls than travel?

Feng Shui Do's

- Ruffled blouses, sequins, and beaded tops are always alluring for nights out in a new town, on the sea, or at a relaxing resort.
- The linear silhouette I describe later remains in play here. Choose long, straight skirts, form-fitting slacks, and—for cool nights out—pair with a slim jacket.
- Long, tight boots (the higher, the better!) and high heels (ditto) are your passports to naughty nocturnal escapades.
- Tulle and chiffon feed the

continued on next page

most closely associated with this zone are the foot, leg, and hip? After all, these are the very bases of our whole body's support. And—best of all—this provides me with the perfect opportunity to discuss one of my favorite subjects: shoes. (Hang on just a bit, fellow shoe queens; that info's coming up soon.) And what could be "hipper"—pardon the pun—than that?

Fashion Profile

Footloose and fancy free! This is your fashion philosophy for the strategic zone.

When it comes right down to it, all of Feng Shui Chic is strategic. As I'm sure you've already deduced, that's what this whole system is about—consciously selecting your clothes and accessories to help achieve a given outcome. And this is just about the most strategic dressing imaginable, don't you think? Like Dorothy in *The Wizard of Oz*, you'll be able to click your heels three times and follow the yellow brick road to the land of your dreams. (And with a little luck and a lot of strategic sense, those heels you're clicking will be Blahniks, baby!)

Here's where the foot metaphor comes into play. You'll be tickled to learn that the Chinese ideogram for foot is the same for the word *virtue*. Your foot, therefore, is the body part that links your highest spirit to all that you desire in life. It stands to reason, then, that by gaining

flow for a cruise to remember. Match these with stretch fabrics for a give-and-take that lets you expand into delicious new directions.

• Map motif accessories rule! By carrying a globe keychain, atlas-patterned towel, or even a mini-map of your hometown in your purse, you are setting the stage for expansion, adventure, and terrific travel wherever you go.

firm footing—physically and spiritually—you pave the way for the very balance that helps you be your most strategic self.

The foot has immense meaning in all of Chinese thought. First and foremost is the purely physical fact that our feet tell us exactly where we are going at any given time. Even more interesting is the metaphor at work here: Firm footing actually establishes our place, our foothold, in society. By now, I'm sure you see exactly why this zone is one of my personal favorites and one of the most important ones for us to honor and use in our daily lives.

You may be amazed to learn that, in ancient China, footprints were actually used as a motif in women's clothing. Footprints have long been thought to represent female energy, which lends a nice yin-yang counterpoint to this zone (remember, the governing force is that of male energy). In addition, wearing footprints as a fashion motif was said to help the wearer gain the foundation needed to make the wisest strategic choices in life.

SOLE FOOD

Whether you're on the road or tripping down familiar pavement, your shoes provide more support than anything else you wear. And I can't help but call this section "sole food" since I've yet to meet the woman whose spirit didn't soar with a divine new pair of shoes. Feng shui teaches us to choose shoes that support us and keep us steady on our paths in super style.

Feng Shui Do's

- Straps provide security and support in casual and dress-up situations.
- For the conservative office, full-back shoes provide the support you need.
- Jeweled shoes are the strategic choice when you want your evening to be a gem.
- Red shoes of any kind fire up energy with loved ones old and new.
- Ballet shoes let you dance into the circle of life when-

continued on next page

SILHOUETTE

Aux armes, soldats! The sleek, chic line of a French military outfit is your cry to fashion battle for strategic Feng Shui Chic. (Is it just me, or is the form-fitting uniform of a French legionnaire one of the sexiest looks ever? If I were on a battlefield and saw one of these *beaux mecs,* I'd surrender in minutes flat. And I could go anywhere in the beautifully tailored suits that Frenchwomen in the armed services wear.)

The good news is that you don't have to be French to look like a million bucks or to reap the rich rewards of Feng Shui Chic dressing for this zone. It's a variation on the classic, tailored look we saw in the creative zone, but with an important twist: Instead of the cinched-in, form-fitting waist that was key there, this zone favors a more elongated look that I like to call a "linear silhouette." Think of Sharon Stone's sleek (yet never cinched) suits, and you get the very pretty picture. Adopt this look yourself, and be prepared to win every strategic battle you enter . . . and then some!

Feng Shui Do's:

- A well-cut trouser paired with a sleek (not over-sized!) jacket and tailored blouse provide you with power for the workplace. Pair these with tight boots— as high as you dare—and you *are* the warrior at work.
- Shiny buttons on your blazer tell the world you're buttoned-up for success.
- A body-conscious, body-hugging dress lets you achieve the recognition you deserve. Pair this with a tight leather jacket for after-hours antics and a deliciously louche effect. It's a look I love: The union of the basic with the luxu-rious, and it creates a yummy yin-yang fashion stance.
- Cigarette pants smoke! Pair these with stilettoes (never clunky Doc Marten–

ever and wherever you choose.
- Sandals and thongs provide open-air support and get you in touch with the natural world.
- Loafers are everyone's best friend on calm country walks.
- Chunky heels announce a modern sophisticate's place in the world.

Feng Shui Don'ts

- High heels are perfect when pleasure seeking, but they create an unbalanced energy in any workplace (though I realize they may be de rigueur if your workplace is onstage in Las Vegas!).
- Scuffed or worn-out shoes reflect scars on your soul.
- Slippers and slide shoes are not office wear. Too-casual footwear results in a slip-pery—even slipshod—atti-tude at work.
- Pointed shoes are like dag-gers: They're great swords for power, but dangerous when love energy's your goal.

type shoes) and add a slim-line cardigan that shows off all your curves.
- Tuxedo and other long, body-conscious skirts work wonders in this zone, especially in the fabrics you'll discover below.

Feng Shui Don'ts

- Flowing skirts and dresses are the antithesis of the sleek, chic silhouette favored in this zone. Remember: You're getting back to basics to launch a super strategy for success.
- Avoid dresses that have elasticized or ribbed waists. Abandon the cinched-waist look of the creative zone when you step into strategic mode.
- Pleated pants are also out, as they tend to draw attention to the waist. Instead, a long, sleek silhouette is what you're after here.
- Crossover straps cause conflict and should be assiduously avoided in this zone.

COLORS

As you can see, I'm giving you fewer color bests here than in other zones. That's because the strategic zone is all about paring down to the essence. Once you get down to basics, you're ready to soar to new heights in all areas of your life.

Feng Shui Do's

- White, for intuition
- Blue, for financial success
- Yellow, for clarity and intellect
- Blue and yellow in any combination, for financial success
- White and yellow, for a real surge of power

Complement these zone colors with your best element shades for fabulous Feng Shui Chic.

Feng Shui Don'ts

- Never wear all white, as this creates a lack of focus—the very opposite of what we seek in the strategic zone.
- I know it's classic downtown chic, but you should avoid wearing an all-black outfit when you need to be at your most strategic. All-black ensembles drain your energy; and good strategy needs good chi/good energy. If you do choose a black-based outfit, be sure to add a splash of color—especially the powerful yellow—to achieve the beauteous balance you seek.

FABRICS

Since the hip is one of the body parts aligned with strategy, you need no further excuse to be hip . . . hipper . . . hippest in this zingy zone.

Feng Shui Do's

- Silk and wool help you weave your way into any social scene.
- Hot new fabrics like bonded knits and metallic threads provide support for heart and soul.
- Natural fabrics—especially linen, cotton, and gabardine—offer the support you need for social success.
- Tropical-weight knits, at the right time of year (or almost anytime of the year if you live in the Sun Belt) provide life structure with a healthy dose of the flexible feel we can always use.

Feng Shui Don'ts

- Faux or man-made materials are big-league no-nos here. In this zone, we get down with what is real—and that means our fashion fabrics, too.

Strategy: The Support Zone | **125**

PATTERNS

Now that you've gotten down to basics, you can help see the big picture with strong, bold prints. March into motion with jungle motifs, which evoke strategic success.

For a conservative workplace, I suggest body-lengthening prints like pinstripes, which also impart strategic strength; why do you think so many bankers wear this as their armor of choice?

Feng Shui Do's

- Jacquard, for firing up, firming ideas
- Twills, for nurturing
- Batik, for tribal
- Abstracts, for new thoughts
- Botanicals and florals, for flowering success
- Pinstripes, for intuition and knowledge

Feng Shui Don'ts

- Wavy and zigzag designs, which create unfocused energy
- Checks and other tiny patterns (but a large, op-art check works because it imparts a bold frame of mind)

ACCESSORIES

Feng Shui Do's

- Tigers, for empowerment
- Flowers, for romance
- Bears, for courage
- Angels, to support those you love
- Coins, for protection

Feng Shui Don'ts

- Arrows, which cut off friendship and support
- Anchors, which weigh you down
- Trees, which here show a play for power, not growth

Zangtra Mind Journal and Ritual

Open the door to opportunity! That's your zangtra theme for this zone.

In Chinese, the symbol for opportunity is two-sided. It reflects both a blockage or impediment . . . and the warrior's skill in creating opportunities and opening new doors. I want you to be in the same winning mind-set.

Understanding is the key to all your opportunities in life. When you are angry or anxious, you are unwittingly closing the doors to all kinds of wonderful options. So by opening your mind, you are taking the most important step to strategic prowess in all areas of your life. Don't forget that expansion is a key theme here.

To achieve this, I ask you to discard all

- preconceived notions of who you are and what you can and cannot do
- demands on yourself and others
- judgments of yourself and others
- the idea of one fixed notion of achievement and success

Be present in the moment, and focus on what's going on right now. How can you be strategic (or beautiful) if you're stewing about something in the future or past?

Light a yellow candle in the quiet place of your choice. Relax, take in a deep breath, and exhale. Feel your breath—and remember what I told you earlier in this chapter about the power of breath and chi. Recite the following blessing:

Strategy: The Support Zone | **127**

I stand with my body planted
Solidly upon the earth
And the spiritual life of Heaven
Fills my heart
And illuminates my spirit
I light my feng shui yellow candle
To help manifest harmony
And balance my life
Illuminating my pathway to create Heaven on Earth

In your journal, identify what makes you angry, sad, and frustrated. Then write down what brings you the most fulfillment and joy. One client, Shamika, wrote:

- My kids
- Parts of my job
- My church
- Reading
- Travel

Sometimes, we feel much better merely identifying those things that give us joy, especially when we promise ourselves to incorporate these people or activities more fully into our life. Joy is a powerful promoter of good chi, and that in turn puts us into our most efficient strategic mode.

Next, list those things that trigger negative thoughts and emotions—and propose practical solutions.

Shamika wrote:

- Most of my job . . . continue searching for a new one
- My boyfriend, much of the time . . . ditto!
- My mother . . . lay boundaries so that we can improve our relationship
- My diet . . . buy only healthy foods from now on

You get the picture. Merely by identifying those things or people that caused her stress and strife, Shamika took a healthy—and very strategic—first step toward eliminating the negatives in her life.

To bring this full circle, once again promise yourself to spend more time on those things that bring you happiness.

One last, but super-important, tip: Doing volunteer work will expand your horizons and will remind you that, no matter how bad your present situation may be, there are always folks who are worse off.

ZANGTRA EXERCISE
1. Sit on the floor in a comfortable position.
2. Close your eyes and visualize the color yellow.
3. Feel the warmth of this color, beginning at your navel and traveling throughout your body and up to your head.
4. Now, feel the color orange, which contains essential earth energy, and accept it in all parts of your body. Let this nurturing energy relax you, purify you, and balance you with nature and yourself.

In this calm state, you are now ready for the body exercise itself.
1. Stand up and bring your knees together.
2. Bring your feet so close together that they touch.
3. Place the knuckles of your left hand over your right hand and extend the hand fully, away from your body.
4. In so doing, you are bringing your warrior's sword upward to the sky.
5. Visualize your blade perfectly aligned with your body and soul.
6. With one swift action, lower your sword in front of you.

In this swift, sure movement, you are opening your door to opportunity and choice. You are the strategic warrior, and the warrior is you.

If the Shoe Fits

Strategically minded shoppers should choose shoes not only to match their handbags but also to attract the energy they need to cross the finish line first (and in style, of course).

Association	Color	Fabric	Pattern	Toe shape	Heel shape
Creativity	Black, indigo	Brocade, quilted, washed	Asymmetrical, waves	Curved, open toe	Slides, clog, platform
Power	Red, green, purple	Silk, leather	Check, logos, leaves	Square	Low heel wedge, boot
Action	Blue, red	Silk, velvet	Triangle, stars, logos	Pointed	Tapered, high, pump, boot
Balance	Tan, beige, brown	Suede, leather, canvas	Round, floral	Square	Flat, sneaker, ballet
Wisdom	Silver, gray, copper, gold	Leather, silk	Rectangle, sculptural	Curved, closed toe	Sling back, curved

Mama's Got a Brand-New Bag

Association	Color	Fabric	Pattern	Style
Creativity	Indigo, black	Brocade, washed	Asymmetrical, waves	Horizontal, clutch
Power	Green, purple, red	Straw, bamboo, woven	Leaves, logos	shoulder bag, handles
Action	Blue, red, orange	Silk, velvet	Stars	Jeweled, sparkles
Balance	Yellow, brown, orange	Leather, suede	Flowers, fauna	Round, backpack, pouchy
Wisdom	Silver, gold	Metallic	Rectangle	Fluted, oval

Knowledge: The Big

Picture Zone

KOAN
"Real knowledge is not found in knowing, but in doing."

ZONE OM
"Saying 'no' is to know."

ZONE OM TIP
Zap your zone om onto your backpack, briefcase, or PDA for a real information injection.

COLORS | Lavender, blue, yellow
SILHOUETTE | Classic, boxy Jackie O–shaped
BODY | Hip, leg

Zone Wisdom

This chapter will help teach you how to find knowledge
- within yourself
- in the outside world
- in specific courses of study
- to make the best and wisest choices in your life

Quick: What verb comes to mind when we think about knowledge?

If you guessed "gaining," "getting," or "amassing," you and I think alike. But now I'm going to tell you to throw what you think you know about knowledge right out the window. (Sorry 'bout that, but you'll see why in just a minute.)

It's true, isn't it, that most of us think about getting degrees, taking courses, or amassing knowledge in some way. Yet the zone om here tells us (to paraphrase Nancy Reagan, something I thought I'd never in my life do) to just say no.

I know this takes some getting used to, so let me explain. I certainly don't mean to ask you to jettison everything you've learned through school or life, or to cast away all the life learning that you hold dear to your heart. That said, I remind you that getting back to basics—decluttering, if you will—is a central focus of feng shui, and that's exactly what I'm asking you to do now.

Now, I'm certainly not asking you to forget everything you learned in school, problem-solving skills you've gained on the job, or any of the other great stuff we learn day to day. But I do invite you to discard

- old, ineffective ways of doing things
- stereotypes—including remnants of racism, sexism, or homophobia from your early years
- information fed to us by the media. Say, as my client Karen did: "For the next month, I'm going to read the daily papers and eliminate silly TV shows, supermarket tabloids, and video games from my life." (Turns out Karen turned this into a long-range habit, and she hasn't looked back on to Jerry Springer's show or *The Price Is Right* once!)

I call this taking time out for spiritual R&R. Doing so allows us to relax, restore, and rejuvenate our lives. Some of you may be lucky enough to do this by visiting a spa, retreat, or serene foreign land. Though lovely, none of the above is required. We can achieve the same renewed spirit just by allowing ourselves to clear our minds . . . and allow ourselves to go into ourselves for a period of time.

Some of you may choose to do this by finding the proverbial quiet corner for a half hour every day. Others among you may say, "Carole, I don't have that luxury." To which I respond: "I perfectly understand." If this is the case, the time-outs that you take can be done while waiting in line at a bank, when waiting for your kids to get out of school, or while at your supermarket checkout. The best part is that you don't need to take any special equipment, because your spirit is always with you.

You know how we reset our computers when they freeze or stall? Think of these mini time-outs as your personal "refresh" button. Even the time we spend waiting at traffic lights gives us the opportunity to do just that.

How do you take a time-out? It isn't really all that hard. What I do is

- make a conscious decision that I'm "checking out" for a few minutes. (As many of you know, the body often answers to our mind—telling it what to do rather than to accept what it's telling us is always good medicine.)
- close my eyes and feel my body and its energy. When we do this, most of us first feel some tension in our temples and around our eyes, and then feel other parts of our body from there. Listening to our body is always a good idea, and you'll probably feel a sore shoulder or tired ankle you never knew you had!
- be perfectly still, and let my chi (body energy) re-adjust itself. (You actively help this to happen by sheer dint of taking a time-out.)
- not permit negative thoughts to enter my mind. Banish anger at your boss or envy of your best friend's new BMW before these ideas can take root in your head. Replace them as they occur with

positive power: "I have a good marriage; why should I let anger over a misplaced sock ruin my relationship and my health?" or "Let me be happy for Nancy's success and be glad that, unlike many people on Earth, I have plenty to eat and a car that gets me where I need to go."

If you've been reading every chapter in sequence, you certainly know how important the principle of rooting ourselves is. While some systems of thought call this centering or grounding, feng shui most often uses the term *rooting*. I love this, because it reinforces the highly important notion of being connected to Earth. That's precisely why the leg and hip are the body parts traditionally associated with the knowledge zone.

By making the conscious decision of gifting ourselves with these time-outs—what I call feng shui spiritual times—delivers another gorgeous bonus: It releases us from making instant decisions. Remember what I said in the last chapter about thinking before we act? That strategy is reinforced by the om we learn here. By taking the time to reflect, we are better able to cope with stress because we allow ourselves to balance our bodies and souls to achieve a kind of personal equilibrium. This, in turn, lets us make informed, judicious decisions rather than rash ones—and isn't that what knowledge is all about?

This is *also* what beauty is all about. On one of her more recent albums, Joni Mitchell (whom I love, period) has a line I adore: "Happiness is the best face lift." Amen!

Think there's no correlation between our inner state and the lines on our face? Anyone of you over forty already "gets" this, but I say to you all: There's no doubt this is true. We all know someone whose looks have been touched by tragedy or times of stress and has it written all over their face.

By saying no to stress, as our zone om tells us, we are letting go—and so we are able to receive, rather than react. By permitting ourselves to receive, we don't go into immediate reaction mode; and I

THE POWER TO
KNOW "NO"

Knowledge is power . . . but only if we use it wisely and well.

It's never easy to make major changes in our lives, but it is possible—especially if we acknowledge our intent through feng shui. In large part, this comes from knowing when to say "no," or to move on to a new stage of your life. Recall, if you will, that decluttering our life is a stepping-stone to knowledge; this includes getting rid of relationships or habits that are toxic or just plain don't work.

- To bring an end to any cycle of events in your life—an old job or house—or to signal the end of any habits you want to break, wear clear quartz or a silver moon crescent as earrings or a brooch, or dazzlingly dangling from a charm bracelet or necklace.
- To say sayonara to a bad relationship, avoid blue rib-

continued on next page

don't have to tell you that when we're stressed, pressed, or suppressed is when we're most likely to do or say something we later regret. I've done this, world leaders have done it, and so have you.

This is where the koan and zone om, at first glance contradictory, come together and make perfect yin-yang sense. The koan tells us that we learn from doing, and this is where real knowledge lies. Our zone om, on the other hand, advises us to "just say no." Upon first reading this, you might think that saying no represents the converse of the koan, which tells us to act. Not so! Saying no is very much a conscious act, as philosophers from Confucius to Camus have told us, and it is thus a very active—and, yes, potent—act indeed.

Some of my clients have told me they feel guilty taking time for themselves, or even for the mental process of saying no . . . and this should never be the case. To some extent, this is an outgrowth of the superwoman syndrome, which tells us we have to be all things to all people—and nothing to ourselves. Banish that thought, please. Making space for yourself not only provides the soul the nourishment we need, but actually allows us to be better to people in our lives—friends, lovers, and colleagues alike. Most important of all is that, unless you do take the time to say no, you will never know the only person who will truly let you see the essential: yourself.

bons. In feng shui, this is a sign of mourning—and you know darn' well that, like Mary Richards, you're going to make it after all! Just make sure that the hat you throw up into the air is a yellow one in this zone, and remember that love *is* all around. Knowledge is, too, and it's there for all of us to find.

Darla did exactly that. Like a high-powered lawyer/wife/supermom plucked out of a TV drama or magazine profile, she was killing herself trying to have it all. The result: In the end, she wasn't enjoying a single moment of her life. (If she had her own show, it would have to be called *Stress Central* and star Sela Ward.)

So Darla instituted her very own time-outs. At home, she told her family—including her husband—that one half-hour every night was Darla Time. In the office, she would call a brief, impromptu time-out with her law partners whenever heated debates were going nowhere but straight to Stressville.

In both cases, the result was the same. Just like we clear our computer's cache to make it run more smoothly, Darla's time-outs let her mind and body do the same. After refreshing her soul and spirit, she was able to receive, not just react—and this allowed for smooth sailing in all parts of her life.

This is why "chilling" can be thrilling. By "chilling out," we're able to reconnect with ourselves, and this helps us know others better

KEEPING KNOWLEDGE IN FLOW

The glory of knowledge is not to possess it, but to be able to share it with the world at large. For this reason, consider helping others in your community as a wonderful way to keep knowledge in circulation while making a difference to the world in which we live.

We've already talked about volunteerism in the support zone. There's one major difference between here and there. In that zone, helping others is more of an external push; in this one, it originates from within, and emanates from without. The final outcome, though, is what matters, and that's all about using your newfound knowledge to make the world a better place.

as well. Give yourself permission to refresh your soul and rebuild your spirit. This is the cornerstone to self-acceptance—and with it comes greater knowledge of the world at large.

I'll even go one step further and say that these spiritual time-outs are not elective, but essential. (Think of these breaks as your spiritual beauty rest; it's as restorative as spraying Evian water on your skin during a long flight.) These "spirit breaks" uncover and acknowledge our inner spirit so we can know ourselves . . . and begin to know others, too.

When you're in a reflective mode, I ask you to consider your mind a garden that needs pruning and weeding. Choose what you want and need in life—and what you don't. It's not always an easy task, but it must be done if we are to move forward and cultivate our garden, just as Voltaire long ago said we should.

And above all: Don't let others' thinking cloud your own. The influence of our family and friends can be good, bad, or indifferent, but this is our time to acknowledge and honor our thoughts. They are ours and no one else's. In the same vein, now is not the time to sing the blues by regretting past beliefs, decisions, or acts. Don't sing the blues—wear them! (I mean this quite literally because blue is an integral color for this, the knowledge zone.)

Wearing the Blues

Blue is the color associated with the knowledge zone, so it's no surprise that students spend their school days clad in blue jeans. However, wisdom is also gleaned away from our schoolrooms or offices. Be sure to don the kind of jeans or denim skirt that will attract not only compliments, but also the energy you need to make knowledge work for you.

Association	Silhouette	Finish
Flow	Basic flare, ribbon belts, rips and tears, darts	Stonewash, riverwash, sun faded, streaky
Growth	Classic trouser, pegged leg, slim boot cut	Stretch fabrics, cotton ridge, dark rinse and tints, green tea wash, patches
Action	Slim fit, boot cut flare, flare leg, vent leg, red stitching, stovepipe	Baked finish, crystal beads, logos
Balance	Capri, overalls, wide boot	Sandblast, lightwash, natural, flowers, embroidery
Family	Novelty belts, back leg pleats, zippers, rivets, rear darts, bell-bottoms, slits	Vintage, distressed

Skirting the Issue

Association	Skirt length	Silhouette	Finish/Color
Flow	Ankle	Shirred waist, semi-circular	Colorwash and tints, blues, blacks
Growth	Below knee	Straight line, slit front, back, or side	Natural, florals, embroidery
Action	Mini	Tapered, v-notch yoke, vent	Baked reds, plums, pinks, purple
Balance	Above knee	Natural flare, natural waistband	Vintage, distressed, yellow, tan, khaki, brown
Structure	Mid-calf	Very high or low waist, detailed belt, straight with inverted pleat	Acid wash, orange, white, autumn tones

This all having been said, we need not just to think about, but to use the knowledge we gain. That's where the koan comes into play. Only by acting on our newfound knowledge can we truly know. It's by doing—by improving ourselves, our families, and our communities— that we can shape our knowledge and learn even more. And, while book learning is also important (it would be hard to erect a building without studying physics), it's only by combining the real world with academic pursuits that we really make knowledge work for us. In a phrase: Knowledge is the beauty of education and the pleasure of discovery. Or, as Saint-Exupéry wrote: *On ne voit bien qu'avec le cœur. L'essentiel est invisible pour les yeux.* (We only see clearly with our hearts. That which most matters is invisible to our eyes.)

Several years ago, my husband and I traveled to France. At the urging of my dear friend Sandy, we made a special sidetrip to Mont-Saint-Michel. Set high on a promontory, and usually engulfed by fog, this is a mystical and marvelous place, one that is widely recognized as the spiritual center of France. Its history tells us why. After the exhumed body of a bishop was found to have fingerprints on its head, Christians the world over believed them to be the touch of angels who had visited the site.

This apparent miracle is commonly interpreted as symbolizing that the priest's—and all of our—spirits are always safe, everlasting, and protected by God. Thus do I believe that the souls of all of those who perished in the World Trade Center, in Pennsylvania, and at the Pentagon are eternal.

But what, exactly, is the connection between the spirit and knowledge? In China and many other Asian countries, it is believed that ancient spirits (sometimes called sages) actually provide us with knowledge. Their spirit embraces not only everlasting life, but the wisdom of the ages. By listening to the spirits that are everywhere—either at an acknowledged holy place, like a Shinto shrine, or on Mont-Saint-Michel—we allow ourselves to be open to the knowledge that is all around us that asks to be gleaned. As I said earlier, knowledge is not only about book learning, but about learning to be open to the wisdom the universe can provide us.

I invite you, with all my heart, to climb the symbolic stone steps to Mont-Saint-Michel and learn how to harness the power of knowledge in your own life.

Fashion Profile

You say you've always wanted to look like Jackie O? Rejoice, girlfriends, 'cuz now's your big chance!

The beautiful, boxy suits that Oleg Cassini designed for this cherished first lady are your style guideposts here. Uncluttered, unfettered, and totally fabulous is how you want to dress in the knowledge zone. I think this is much more than a charming coincidence since Mrs. Onassis, who very easily could have led a pampered, self-involved life, thirsted for knowledge instead. From foreign languages to political science, from literature to the history of art, this was a lady who wanted to expand her mind and know her world in every way she could.

When should you use your feng shui finest? When you
- need to call upon your utmost brainpower—for instance, before taking a hard test or while studying for a professional license
- are looking within yourself for self-knowledge at a particularly difficult personal period
- seek new direction in life and need to summon all the knowledge in your arsenal to make the right choice

SILHOUETTE
In the knowledge zone, square means flair! Yes, the classic boxy look of Jackie O or Brooks Bros.–type suits works wondrously well. Happily, though, the circle is also a very important shape in this zone, which means that you can add visual verve to this silhouette, especially when stepping out after the sun goes to its sleepy bed.

Feng Shui Do's

- A square-cut Grace Kelly–type gown is fabulous feng shui when paired with a rounded stole or shawl—faux fur, if you please.
- A rectangular top worn with a circular skirt
- Go Garbo with square, wide-legged pants and a square-shouldered sailor's blouson.
- A square-cut evening dress topped with a round-shouldered jacket makes you a fashion force with great feng shui.
- On a cold winter's day, face the world with lioness leggings worn under a funky balloon skirt—very Cyndi Lauper retro chic!—but

make sure to pair this with a square-cut jacket for the yin-yang square-and-rectangle shapes for this zone.

Feng Shui Don'ts

- Tapered, sleek looks make you stiff and unreceptive to your thoughts and to those of others.
- Fight fashion flotation! Billowing skirts or dresses make you uncertain, unfocused, and undecided. They're the very antithesis of the boxy silhouettes that help you get rooted here.

COLORS

When should you wear your knowledge zone colors? Whenever you need to reap wisdom and call upon all of life's lessons. For instance, when you
- take an especially important exam
- are studying super-challenging material
- need to be your absolute wisest—say, when dealing with a touchy family issue or personal dilemma

Feng Shui Do's

- Yellow, for power and wealth
- Lavender, for the spirit you need to realize your dreams
- Orange, for the mind boost to bring you success in all endeavors
- Peach, for health, happiness, and peachy-keen ideas
- Yellow, aqua, and blue are the perfect combination for this zone. By combining the sand, sea, and earth, you invite all the world's knowledge into your life.

Feng Shui Don'ts

- Black, which deflects decisions. Avoid wearing this color when strong actions or decisions are required in your life.

Knowledge: The Big Picture Zone | **143**

- Black plus blue equals a bruised you. Always avoid this color combo, especially when mind expansion's your goal.

FABRICS

Soft, comfortable fabrics are your launching pad to the knowledge you seek. This is because they allow you to focus on freeing your mind, not being a slave to contour and fashion. Soft is smart in the knowledge zone!

Feng Shui Do's

- Taffeta, for adventure
- Chiffon, to capture your goals
- Lace, to show you're both naughty and nice
- Tulle, for festive flair
- Tweed, to show you're "countrified" and down-to-earth
- Flannel, to invite snuggling
- Velvet, for sensuality
- Silk gabardine, for smooth sailing in all that you do
- Pre-washed denim, to show you can stand up to anything

Feng Shui Don'ts

- Unwashed denim results in fuzzy, unfocused energy—not smart!
- Shetland wool, too coarse to allow you to accumulate knowledge smoothly

PATTERNS

In this zone, the patterns you wear are ever so important—and the ones you don't, even more so. Invite wisdom into your life by optimizing feng shui with the motifs recommended below.

Feng Shui Do's

- Stripes, to increase knowledge
- Jacquard, to cultivate clarity
- Tahitian and Balinese patterns, to invite wisdom from all points of the globe

Feng Shui Don'ts

- Checked patterns, which create unstable energy and dissuade new thought patterns from entering your life
- Houndstooth may be mod, but it can also make you dizzy—and what's further from smart than that?

ACCESSORIES
Fruit and fish find you freedom of thought in the knowledge zone!

Feng Shui Do's

- Bells illuminate your high ideals and let freedom of expression ring.
- Fruit motifs herald abundance in all areas of your life, including the intellectual.
- Fish patterns as charms and pins find you swimming in wealth.
- Swags represent happy, smiling faces—wear more than three strands for optimal effect.

Feng Shui Don'ts

- Arrows pierce and thus fragment knowledge.
- Jagged, sharp, asymmetrical patterns separate linear lines and thus cogent thought.

The zangtra steps for this zone teach us how to lay the foundation from which to grasp as much knowledge and understanding as we can, in all areas of our lives. Introspection paves the way for self-respect. Then, when self-love and self-understanding are directed outward, we are able to allow truth to flow into our lives. And always remember that Chinese mystics tell us that healing is nothing more or less than standing in truth.

Get comfortable and relax your mind so that you are able to tap into your inner reservoir.

- Journal all your present feelings, from the most positive to the most negative.
- List your fears and joys. By doing so, you are making strong inroads to acceptance—the most fundamental facet of self-knowledge.
- Go for your goals. This could be success in a university extension course or the wisdom to fix a problem you're having with a colleague or friend. Visualize yourself three days, three weeks, and three months from now. This will help you set simple goals; structure them; and achieve them.
- Accept the knowledge that who you are is who you should be . . . where you are in life is where you should be . . . and that you are growing and learning as the universe intends you to.
- Know that knowledge is not a fixed entity, but grows and changes along with you—and that you use the knowledge you gain in life to show yourself the path of light at all times in your life. Sometimes, we think we know it all. But feng shui tells us to be open to accepting new knowledge and learning as it comes into our life: to learn new ways and travel new roads as they are shown to us.

As you journal, you will begin to notice that everything you create becomes part of a larger movement toward a goal. Feng shui teaches us to move in a full circle from one zone to the next. This helps us create balance and confidence—and ultimately, when we bare the truth at the root of our lives, boundless joy. By acknowledging the internal (your mind), you are stimulating action in the external world. Root for yourself—and root yourself—and the knowledge you seek in your life will flow to you—today, tomorrow, and in all the days to come.

ZANGTRA EXERCISE

As a friend of mine said: "The day pigs fly, I'll hear a bowl that sings." Well, I still haven't seen a flying pig, but I *have* seen a bowl that sings!

Let me introduce you to the singing bowl. It is a unique device, typically crafted of bronze or glass, which has been used in the East for centuries—and it is a wonderful way to connect yourself to healing sounds. As stress busters go, I can recommend these beautiful bowls with heart and soul. Where to buy them? At spiritual bookstores—and I'm glad to say there's one in almost every town nowadays.

There are many types of these bowls available. How to choose the one that's best for you? Try them out first; most stores won't mind if you do. You'll want to consider the aesthetic considerations of color and size, of course, but even more important is the sound these bowls make. You'll be surprised to learn how different each one sounds. Choose the bowl whose sound is most harmonious to your own ears.

Use your singing bowl whenever you seek inspiration or deep relaxation. Here's how to do it.
- Hold the bowl gently in your hands.
- Place your mouth near the upper rim.
- Sound the word "om," listening to the sound as it travels over the

rim and throughout your body, and vibrates toward the outside world.

- Repeat the om chant for several minutes, or until you feel your whole body relax into blissful serenity. This is the first step toward the healing you seek.
- Notice how the sounds you create affect your body—pay special attention to involuntary sensations of movement and body temperature.
- Remember: Practice makes perfect. As you experiment with your singing bowl, you will begin to learn which of your chants helps you most.

This exercise reinforces one of the key messages of this chapter: By listening, you are gaining the receptivity that is the foundation of all knowledge. I saw this work firsthand with my client and friend, Alexa. A major type-A personality, Alexa was always on the go—work, social life, travel—and never seemed to enjoy a minute of any of it. What's more, she chatted so much to others that she never seemed to listen to herself. I asked her to get two singing bowls—one for her office and one for her home. She did so begrudgingly, yet "om'd" her bowl twice daily as instructed. "I don't know how this works," Alexa admitted, "but it does. It's a kind of forced time-out for me, and it actually does center me and calm me down. It also makes me hear the sound of my own voice, which is helpful because I'm now able to tell when I'm talking too much!" I promise your singing bowl will work exactly the same wonders for you.

CHAPTER ELEVEN

Health:

The Harmony Zone

KOAN

"No matter how tall the mountain, it cannot block out the sun."

ZONE OM

"Take one step at a time and you can climb the highest hill."

ZONE OM TIP

Paste your zone om on your medicine cabinet, on your gym bag, or on a vitamin carrier in your purse or attaché.

COLORS | Green, blue
SILHOUETTE | Minimalist: smooth, sleek,
and straight ahead
BODY | Arm; this is also the zone
most closely related to chi,
or breath

Zone Wisdom

This chapter will teach you how to
• take the time to breathe for optimal chi (the very cornerstone of optimal health)

- learn to listen to your body—and what it is telling you
- restore your body's equilibrium through zangtra exercise
- think positively, thus acknowledging the connection beween our minds and health

Zone Profile

Come enter the zone of the blue dragon, perhaps the most powerful life area of all.

Why the "blue dragon"? Because Chinese legend tells us that this is the dragon of spring, who represents the healing energies of breath and air. You already know that, in the Chinese language, breath and chi share the same symbol. So you'll certainly understand how the healing imagery of the air that we breathe is integral to our overall health.

Throughout this book, I've tried to Westernize the tenets of feng shui to make you feel comfortable, so that you'll readily understand how these fit into your daily life. But the legend of the blue dragon is just too delicious to resist, so forgive me for indulging myself—and you—in this wondrous tale.

The blue dragon is believed to arise in spring as a potent symbol of regeneration and rebirth. But that's just the start. More metaphorically, this dragon symbolizes the union of the upper body (expression) and the lower torso (abundance). This unique yin-yang union of imagination and rhythmic force provides us with the power we need to transform our lives into abundance in all areas—especially in the realm of health.

In art, the blue dragon is portrayed as rising from the depth of the sea to the heavens above. As he does so, he fills the vast universe with harmony and turns darkness to light. At the same time, the blue dragon bridges heaven and earth, filling the whole world with his benevolent energy.

As he travels through the universe, the blue dragon blesses us with his healing energy. And here we come to a very important point: The power to affect our health lies in our very own hands. The blue dragon bestows his gifts upon us mortals, but it's up to us to use them wisely and well.

This, I think you'll agree, is in marked contrast to the traditional Western idea of health, which lies in treating a given symptom with medicines, surgeries, and pills. In the East (and here I mean not just China, but in nearly all Far Eastern lands) general wellness is a far more important goal. Individual symptoms—a sore throat, blurry vision, fatigue—occur when our chi is poorly aligned . . . and this comes from disrespecting our bodies and refusing to acknowledge preliminary warning signs when they occur.

So I caution you: Watch out for burnout! This isn't a mathematical equation; your body will tell you when you are feeling run-down, overtired,

MUSIC: NATURE'S OWN MEDICINE

Natural healers have long sung the praises of music as a healing force. Now, researchers at the nation's most prestigious medical schools have conducted laboratory trials and proved this to be true. When our mind is serene, spirited, and sanguine, our health follows suit.

I think of music as nature's medicine. It lifts us up when we are down, raises our spirits when we need a little inspiration, and conjures up nostalgic times and the promise of distant lands.

Take your own little "music for health" break by

- keeping a Walkman or CD player in your desk at work.
- designating family music times once or twice a week.
- attending concerts or other live performances as often as you can.

My own favorites are Debussy's "Claire de lune" and Atlantis's

continued on next page

New Age "Crystal Cave." My co-author, David, loves the soothing sounds of Irish folk singer Luka Bloom. Why not make your own personal date with whatever healing music makes *your* spirit soar— and start the healing process as you do?

or just generally stressed. And it is up to you, and you alone, to feel your body's signals, respect them, and do whatever necessary to realign your chi.

I understand that this can be difficult. Some of us have greater luxuries of time and money than others; and if we have children, our own needs seem to be thrust somewhere very far away. Yet, just as I told you in the previous chapter about personal time-outs, so too do you need to monitor your own health. By taking the time to breathe, we acknowledge our body's needs. Breathing actually allows us to take things one step at a time, which is the very message of this zone's om.

When we do this, we adjust our chi, and can put our bodies back into first gear. After all, we realign our cars' tires; doesn't it make perfect sense that we would respect our own bodies in the very same way?

My client Janese did just that, especially after I used the car metaphor with her. "Good God, Carole!" she exclaimed. "When you put it that way, I feel like a fool. Do you know that I take much better care of my car than my body? I'm a maniac about getting those 10,000-mile tune-ups, oil changes, and all the rest. But do you know how long it's been since I saw a dentist? At least two years! And forget about yoga and all that other stuff. That's fine for Madonna, but I have two kids, a husband, and a nonstop career. I realize that my body is as important as my car, but where do I find the time?"

I told Janese, perhaps a bit more sternly than usual, that she had to *make* the time. Breathing is key, and the zangtra exercises you'll find in this and other chapters can be done at your desk or workplace, even if you take just minutes out of your day. By the same token, nearly every city and suburb has a salon or studio offering fifteen-minute chair massages, usually for as little as a dollar a minute. While not as beneficial as a full body massage, a deep-tissue attack on your neck and shoulders can leave you feeling incredibly refreshed, realigned, and ready to take on the world. And if your company has an in-house gym, do make use of it, even if it's for just fifteen minutes a day to start.

That's precisely what Janese did, starting slowly and building to a thirty-minute workout each day. She also began to have weekly massages ("My therapist says he's never felt shoulders as tense as mine," Janese admitted), and after only a few months, Janese felt and looked like a new person. "The combination of body-work and working out was pivotal for me—it's almost like I'm pummeling the stress out of my body and banish-

THE HEALING POWER OF BATHS

We all know that nothing beats a warm, leisurely bath in terms of beating stress. In today's busy times, we regard lolling in the suds as a special personal treat . . . but in ancient Rome, baths were both a social ritual and rite of health. If you haven't turned on to the pleasure of a bath brimming with essential oils, now's your chance.

In the blue dragon zone, the following scents work best:

- Lemongrass
- Bamboo
- Sandalwood (men love this one, I promise!)
- Your favorite floral aroma—rose and lilac are especially known for their healing powers

While bathing, let your mind move to waterfalls, breezes, and the scent of spring. Tickle your senses, de-stress your body, and

continued on next page

Health: The Harmony Zone | **153**

soothe your soul with a scented bath. Regain the equilibrium you need for heightened health.

ing it from my psyche as well."

Taking it one step at a time is key to our health—and, indeed, to all aspects of our lives. (Remember the old adage that "only fools rush in"?) It's equally important that we rid ourselves of the emotional and physical baggage that can affect our chi—and our health. The following example, taken from my own early days as a feng shui apprentice, illustrates this principle most clearly.

As my master and I ascended a mountain on the outskirts of Hong Kong, I heard him call: "Carole, what did you take with you this morning to prepare yourself for the climb?" I turned to him and replied (feeling totally prepared with the right answer): "Water." "Anything else?" he asked. I laughed and said, "Certainly not."

Master Leung signaled to me to stop at that point, and we found a rock to relax on. At that moment, he asked me, "When you hike, where do you look? At the side of the mountain, or down at the trail?" I thought for a moment, then replied: "I look forward."

"Exactly!" my master cried. "Never look down or back, Carole. Learn to look ahead, and to focus only on your present path. This teaches you to light your own way, and to lead yourself on the road of life. It also shows us that we cannot ascend a mountain while carrying baggage. Carrying mental or physical baggage—or both— will only burden us and hinder our ascent to the mountaintop."

So, friends, I ask that just as I did, you take the first step toward letting go of the baggage you carry in this life. It takes courage and concentration to do it, but it can—and should—be done. The blue dragon shows us the way, through the powers of change that he has bestowed upon us all. Call upon the strength, vibrancy, and benevolent healing in the universe to attain your own ascendance and to take charge of your own healing.

Take one step at a time, and remember the wisdom of your health koan: Even the tallest mountain can't block out the sun. The power to restore our chi and to enjoy optimal mental and physical health has been provided by the blessed blue dragon. His power is all around us, just waiting to nourish our bodies and souls.

Fashion Profile

This zone's fashion forecast isn't about flourish and fantasy, but about clean, simple, healthy lines. When the hippies in the musical *Hair* exhorted us to "Let the Sun Shine In," they knew what they were talking about! Can you think of a better image for the wellness zone? (And it reflects the koan nearly perfectly, too.)

Yes, in the health zone, minimalism is a major fashion stance. Forget the fanfare; your goal here is to keep things basic to set the stage for the chi you cherish. An unadorned, yet always chic, vertical silhouette clears the pathways of our body's chi, and keeps your mind and spirit as fresh as a daisy. Best of all is that these simple lines help us travel light—one step at a time, just as our zone om tells us to do.

SILHOUETTE

Always wanted to be a flapper? Tootsie, your time is now! This is the place where a spaghetti-strapped, straight-line dress makes you the most alluring creature in the world.

A sleek, slender silhouette rules this zone, and Calista Flockhart is its goddess. No one looks more smashing in straight, uncluttered lines, whether it be slacks or a skirt, and whether she pairs it with a classic-fit sweater or button-down shirt. Think of the long line of the bamboo stalk—strong, prosperous, and at peace with the world. That's your fashion mantra in the important health zone.

Feng Shui Do's

- A sexy slip dress, for a healthy dose of romance
- Tube dresses or skirts, which combine linear energy with body-conscious allure
- A strapless dress, cut as deep as you dare—but with a straight silhouette, not a billowing or cascading skirt
- A dropped-V waistline makes a beautiful bridal dress and assures fertility and a lifetime of health
- A miniskirt or dress, if your legs are lovely, which complements the straight lines of this zone with the za-zoom you desire
- A shift dress—think Talbots here—is perfect to signal quiet authority at work while honoring the health zone
- A trumpet dress, your bugle call to move forward in life—beautifully, boldly, and in perfect health

Feng Shui Don'ts

- Rips and tears are the very antithesis of the unbroken lines you need for terrific health zone chi. You may be a survivor, but you're not on the TV show—so stop dressing like you are in the middle of a rescue mission!
- Wraparound or billowing skirts create unstable energy in this zone and can negatively impact your general health. These are no-nos, Nanette.
- Jagged edges—on your pants, skirt, or anywhere else—destroy both your personal harmony and your body's chi. Please avoid!

COLORS

It should come as no surprise that blue and green are your most healthful hues—hospitals and wellness centers use these colors to soothe patients and staff. These are the colors of meadows, the sea, and the sky . . . the very symbols of serenity and calm, they set the stage for glorious health.

Color your spirits with nature's crayons! The health zone's colors are those of spring. As bright and beautiful as an aster bloom, they signal new beginnings, abundance, and rebirth—as fine for the soul as they are for fashion.

Feng Shui Do's

- Green, for harmony and health
- Blue, for timeless vision, expansion, and calm. (Blue is also the chi color for life and symbolizes oxygen—a prerequisite to gentle healing.)
- Golden brown, for nurturing
- Peach, for fire energy's warmth and health
- Lavender, to clear the thoughts and spirit

Feng Shui Don'ts

- White, which destroys health and harmony
- Black and gray, which create an emotional overload and disharmony—and bad chi means bad health
- Red, which provides a feverish energy
- Violet, which can cause depression

FABRICS

Go ahead, make Bruce Springsteen's day: In the health zone, we should all be "Jersey girls." Easy, comfortable fabrics are your fashion footnotes for the health zone. Fabrics that breathe, and let *you* breathe, mean fabulous fashion and terrific chi.

Health: The Harmony Zone | **157**

- Chantilly lace or satin, for evening allure
- Chiffon, for a billowy cloud of health
- Flannel, to keep you warm at night
- Silk, to relax your spirit and soul
- Jersey, which lets you relax and revel in life's joys
- Muslin and gauze, for the beach (the perfect place to feel the breath of the sea and regain your own chi)

Feng Shui Don'ts

- Coarse fabrics like unwashed denim or knotty, natural cotton, which create oversensitivity of energy and touch, harmful to both body and soul
- Transparent fabrics form shock waves, which can take their toll on your health

PATTERNS

The pretty pleasures of country-fresh patterns put you in the pink of health in this important zone.

Feng Shui Do's

- Plaids, for longevity
- Tattersall, for luck
- Bamboo prints, for the warmth of the tropics
- Jacquard, for heightened spirit

Feng Shui Don'ts

- Guns and roses, which prohibit peace in your life
- Checks and plaids, which chop off new opportunities for personal expansion

ACCESSORIES

Accessories can do much to balance our energy and restore our chi. My fave raves for this zone help me get through even the tensest (or most tiring) times in perfect health.

Feng Shui Do's

- Flowered scarves, for balanced energy (and turning you into a fashion flower)
- Whistles and bells, to help scare off the bad guys—and their sweet sounds will help you merrily (and healthfully) through life
- Gold-toned belts, brooches—any accessory at all!—will bring the warm, healing rays of the sun to you
- Bow ties and ribbons, to create healthy communication among friends and strangers (Why do you think so many good causes use ribbons as their badges of honor?)

Feng Shui Don'ts

- White, silver, or gray accessories, as they cut off new beginnings and create unstable energy, which never promotes good health
- Metal accessories (other than gold, which lets you glitter in this zone) sever relationships and hinder personal growth
- Jagged-edge and other asymmetrical brooches or belt buckles create disharmony and negatively affect the flow of chi

Zangtra Mind Journal and Ritual

Please allow me to say it one more time: To the Chinese way of thinking, balance is the single most important factor to health. Without balanced chi, our bodies are off-kilter, so feeling—and looking—our best is impossible.

Thus, seeking balance is key. You don't have to actively look for it; just go within your spirit and "walk your talk."

Place a green candle nearby and recite or meditate upon this blessing:

> As I stand and light this flame,
> I invite peace and joy
> to reside in my heart.
> I welcome abundance to my life.
> I renew myself and my vision
> with intent and focus.
> I choose to follow my truth
> nourishing the seeds I have planted
> along the way.
> I celebrate the spiritual riches
> that flow from living in
> Harmony with the Earth.

After reciting or meditating on this blessing, I ask you to consider the following questions as you journal.

- What are the things that unbalance me?
- What do I feel like when I'm unbalanced?
- What is this lack of balance due to?

At the same time, ask yourself these questions.

- How is my body feeling?
- What can I do to feel healthier (exercise, diet, de-stressing, etc.)?

- What bad habits do I need to lose (smoking, alcohol or drug use, overeating)?
- Why are these habits part of my life?
- How can I find the time to regain my chi and respect my body?

Groups like Overeaters or Alcoholics Anonymous teach people not only to respect their bodies, but to begin to understand where their addictions come from. By using your zangtra mind journal as a tool for thought, you too can listen to what your body is telling you, do the best you can for it, and start reaping the rewards of excellent health.

ZANGTRA EXERCISE

This ancient body exercise is based on a simple lotus yoga position called the Rising Spine Motion in Chinese texts. One of the most effective exercises of all, it is used in the Orient to help people heal their wounds—and will help you heal yours.

While not hard to do, this exercise is somewhat more

WELLNESS FOR THE WORLD

Getting in touch with nature is a winning way to make the most of your own health. My favorite ways to do this follow.

- Sow the seeds of health. By planting seeds, you allow new life to blossom and help herald healing new thoughts in your own life. Community gardens, now cropping up everywhere, are the way to go!
- Walk for wellness. Every city sponsors walks to raise money for breast cancer treatment, AIDS awareness, and other good causes. Promote your own health—and that of others—while doing good for your gams.
- Lend a helping hand. Volunteer at a senior citizens' center, read to the blind, or care for a foster child. Do well unto others, and you'll start to feel better than you have in years—guaranteed.

complex than some of the other ones in this book. But take heart, because I promise that once you master this motion, you will begin to see marked improvements in your spirit, chi, and general health. Many of my clients have—and I have, too.

To perform this exercise, follow these steps.

1. Stand upright, with your heels together and feet in an outward, V-formation.
2. Count to ten and breathe in and out slowly.
3. Assume a squatting position with your heels together.
4. Place your arms between your knees, with your fingers extended and touching the floor. (Note: The middle finger energizes the channels of chi and offers support for your whole body.)
5. Keeping your fingertips on the floor and your head down, focus on your middle finger and visualize a lotus in your mind's eye.
6. Inhale and exhale deeply, counting to ten as you do so.
7. Repeat ten times, building to thirty-six sets.

After completing this exercise . . .

1. Stand tall.
2. Raise your heels off the floor slowly.
3. Slowly return your heels to the ground.
4. Repeat twelve times.

Power:

The Abundance Zone

KOAN
"Without an opposing wind, a kite cannot fly."

ZONE OM
"Unless you are pushed, you will not pull."

ZONE OM TIP
Place your zone om on your desk at work or in your home office for all the power you deserve.

COLORS | Aqua, red
SILHOUETTE | Rectangle, square
BODY | Back, neck

Zone Wisdom

This chapter will teach you how to
- acknowledge the importance of power in your life
- appreciate the difference between personal and professional power
- use power wisely and well
- understand that power isn't about ownership— it's about exercising all the options in your life to the fullest and best effect

Power. Of all the zone life areas, this is the one that's the least understood. And since we live in such a power-obsessed culture, it's not hard to see why.

Think about it. Many of the "heroes" our culture reveres are people with power to spare: Sharon Stone (who donates her time and money with the utmost of graciousness) and Donald Trump (who doesn't). But there's a big difference between power and goodness, power and passion, and certainly between power and happiness. Machiavelli may have been majestic, but he surely wasn't munificent!

The message is clear: Power isn't absolute, not what Jean-Paul Sartre would call a *chose-en-soi*. If you think of it this way, your pursuit of power will backfire, because you will ultimately misuse it. Rather, power is a conduit. It's a force you can harness to make the most of your life, but a dangerous thing when used for its own purposes. This is demonstrated by the zone om and koan, which talk about power as a force without which we cannot achieve those things we most desire.

Just as power in its own right is meaningless, so too is power nothing without character. But we can't possess good character unless we first know exactly who we are. That's why finding our true essence—finding what Tao calls our "natural self"—is an absolute requisite for using power well.

How do we do this? It's a lifelong process, and I wouldn't dream of being able to provide you the answer in a paragraph or two. (Now that would be a *real* misuse of the power of the printed word!) But I can tell you how to start.

- Untie the strings of your past, which can hold you back from realizing your dreams. In fact, some folks have umbilical cords so strong that they prevent them from even being able to think about their own dreams, rather than those of their parents.

- Give yourself the love and respect you deserve—even if you haven't been accorded them by your parents, teachers, employers, or other people in your life. Loving yourself gives you the personal power you need to set and achieve your goals in life.

The following story illustrates this point of view.

Keena, whom I met through a client, is proof positive of this. A beautiful and brainy journalist, she was an underachiever, though nobody could understand why she never rose to her fullest potential. Although I'm not a psychologist, I know enough about human nature to see that Keena had been constantly berated by her mother and given no support by her father, who lived in another state. While everyone else looked at her and saw a golden girl, Keena herself never felt quite good

YOUR HEADS UP TO POWER

Want to be the most potent person in the room? Then be a power head with a hat to be reckoned with!

Think it was an accident that Joan Collins made her much-anticipated *Dynasty* entrance with a hat that stretched from here to Timbuktu? Though it was more than a few years ago, I still remember how that grande dame strode into a Denver courtroom with a brim so broad you couldn't even see her eyes till Joan/Alexis lifted it—*when* she wanted to, and *how*.

Prove your power with these top hat choices.

- A Jackie O pillbox, which marries the square shape of this zone with timeless chic
- A square, 40's-era hat—and you can double your power by adorning it with a pin in one of the accessory motifs above

continued on next page

- Baseball caps, which show you're ready to play ball with the best of 'em
- A mannish derby or spectator hat, which portrays a calm, cool, and very collected woman—the very fundamentals of power
- A pith helmet, it shows who's top tiger in the urban jungle—you!

enough—which is why she never achieved the personal success she deserved. Her friend was eventually able to persuade Keena to enter therapy. There, she learned how her childhood had instilled in her a deep fear of failure, as opposed to the I-can-do-anything philosophy someone of her talents deserves. I am happy to say that she is making considerable progress in understanding just how great she really is; in fact, she's presently going after "big" assignments she never would have dared to consider before. "The world is my oyster," is Keena's new motto and mantra. Now that's personal power in its very best form!

- Pull your own strings. Shirley Bassey's classic hit "This Is My Life" is slightly over the top, but truer words were never spoken—or sung. We have only one go-round on this Earth, and it's up to you to decide how you want your time here spent. My friend Paul achieved his parents' dreams by becoming a lawyer, a job at which he was miserable for years. Finally, upon turning forty, he chucked it all and went for a degree in social work, which has been his own dream all along.

In this chapter, you will learn how to use Feng Shui Chic to be the most powerful you that you can be. But because power is such an important force, I do feel the need to provide you with a few last power pointers that I think will serve you well.

- *Power is patience.* Remember that true power—and primo leadership skills—both come from a base of support. (It's no coincidence that Osama bin Laden called his evil empire *Al Qaeda,* which means "the base"—another excellent example of using power for nefarious means.)

- *Power is persistence.* Here again, our zone om and koan serve us well by telling us that power is amassed and strengthened through surviving the gales of opposing forces in life. Once we achieve personal power, we must always strive to maintain its strength and to continue to learn how to use it for positive, uplifting ends.

POWER FLOWERS

Some scents seduce . . . others whisper . . . and a few special aromas shout that you're the boss. Your prime power puss scents:

- Rosemary, for focus and clarity, whatever your aim may be
- Pine, for a long life to the projects you present
- Sage, which clears the air—and lets you get down to business

- *Power is passion.* Having passions in personal and professional areas of our lives is the cornerstone to contentment because it helps us to stay in command. I love the legendary story of how Itzhak Perlman, perhaps the world's greatest violinist, broke a string during a particularly prestigious performance. Rather than stop the concert, he continued to play the piece to its natural end, making concessions to the broken string without interrupting his performance. The moral of the story: When our passion is great enough, it allows us to surmount obstacles, no matter how high they are placed in our path.
- *Power is in people.* Unless we harness power not merely for our own personal goals, but for humanitarian means, all is for naught. Remember what punk poetess Patti Smith sang: "People Have the Power." I pray for you to use the power you gain for the love and life of the people in your own life—and, by creating

good karma, you will also be helping folks you haven't even met. That is power in its very finest hour.

Feng shui also tells us that this is the zone of money and wealth, and that it is. In my practice, as in this book, I prefer to concentrate on the power aspect of this, the abundance zone, because I believe that money comes along with power. But there's an important distinction to be made: There is good and bad money, just as there are good and bad uses of power. When we harness our personal power to make ourselves the very best we can be, financial success will come along for the ride. However, if we try to make money our ultimate goal, we will not succeed—either in making the money we desire or in amassing the kind of power that helps not only ourselves and our loved ones, but all those who are important in our lives.

Most of our perceived heroes happen to be rich, as well as powerful, yet this isn't always a good thing. There's a huge difference between power and wealth that are illusory—say, of a hot hip-hop artist or starlet whose success is based only on looks—and the kind of long-term personal power and enrichment that comes from good works, honing our craft, and helping the world outside with the power we've achieved.

Fashion Profile

Fashion is power, as the fashion mags love to tell us. Whether you seek recognition at work or at play, this is your time to make an entrance in the very grandest style.

Yes, taking center stage is where it's at in this zone. Big, bold, and beautiful looks let you step into the limelight and assure that all eyes are on you. Skirt the issue? Not here you don't! Taking a firm fashion stance demonstrates your power and helps you achieve the success, love, or adventure you so richly deserve.

SILHOUETTE

Come sing the Body Electric when peerless power is what you seek. This is the time to tell your body—in the immortal words of the one and only RuPaul—"You better work!"

You do this in a bit more concerted way in the power zone than in the other life areas we've discussed. Far from a unilateral dressing style, the look for power is all about showing off your body when, where, and how you want. In a phrase, it's all about taking it off, keeping it covered, or doing a little bit of both in order to invite power into your life. Halle Berry is an absolute master of this style, showing off a lot or a little, depending on her aim and intent, and whether the occasion is formal or casual, professional or personal.

Rectangles and squares are the shapes for this zone, but you'll use these forms in anything but a static way. Instead, you can add, subtract, or do a little of both depending on the situation and style you seek.

For this reason, capes are key. Of course, we women hardly need an excuse to make a grand entrance in a cape. Just ask Catherine Deneuve, who can wear this wrap more sensually, powerfully, or haughtily—depending on her objective and mood—than any woman on the planet. (See the tips below to do this with the greatest of ease.)

Feng Shui Do's

- For festival flair or a charity event, wear a cape over a long, narrow skirt.
- For the office, work that cape (pun intended!) over a pair of straight slacks.
- For occasions where you dare to be bare, pair your cape with a short skirt. When you need to seize power, the thigh's the limit!
- A heart neckline proves your power when the recipe is romance.

- Cool your jets. While showing some skin seals your power, too much exposure lets your opinions stream out of control.
- Don't be a basket case. Being too buttoned-up or wearing clothes that are too constricting makes you uptight, not powerful. (Just look at what an excess of Lycra did to *meshuganah* Mariah Carey. Happily, these days she seems to have nixed her sartorial bondage and is doing much better in every possible way.)
- Scruffy shoes give away the power you want to have . . . and hold.
- Owning one good suit is the stuff of Danielle Steele novels, but shows you to be the poor—not powerful—relation in real life.
- Don't box yourself in. Vented jackets let you air your gripes without losing control.
- Pass on the peasant styles. You're a power puss, not a charity case.
- A puffed-out skirt portrays you as full of hot air, not a person of conviction.
- Too-tight pants put you in bondage, not in power.
- Loose clothes of any kind make you a spinning wheel, turning through life without any direction, much less the power you seek.
- Overly starched or pressed clothes don't let you move, and they inhibit flow. You want to wield power, not a steam iron!

COLORS

The vibrant, iridescent colors of nature provide courage—and courage is very much the foundation of power. Wear these hues, and you will connect your soul to your innermost desires and most important intentions.

Feng Shui Do's

- Aqua, for power
- Red, for passion
- Pink, for health—always a prelude to power
- Yellow, for creative flow

Feng Shui Don'ts

- Gray, which promotes negativity, not the positive attitude that goes along with the best use of power
- Scarlet, which creates ethereal, ungrounded energy, not the focus you need
- Metallics, which foster bad health, always out of line with a powerful you

FABRICS
Life is your tapestry, and remember that life is a party—so get ready to shimmy and shake! Let the right fabric choices pave *our* way to power.

Feng Shui Do's

- Leather, for confidence and sex appeal
- Thin wool, to show your assets
- Chiffon, for sheer success
- Velvet, for harmony

Feng Shui Don'ts

- Watered silk, which paints you as limp and drowning—the very obverse of powerful

- Muslin, which gives you a rough time at the company picnic and beyond
- Lycra, which displays all you've got to the world, thus showing your hand and giving away your power
- Metallics (both a color and a fabric), because they cover you with a coat of armor, literally cutting you in half

PATTERNS

Pick your patterns among these potent prints—and amass the personal power you crave.

Feng Shui Do's

- Logos, for prosperity
- Animal prints, for magnetism and strength
- Bold patterns, for elegance and poise, which help paint a picture of personal power
- Flower prints, for happiness (without which power means nothing at all)

Feng Shui Don'ts

- Zigzags put you out of step, thus creating confusion and indecision
- Small gingham prints, which portray you as ungrounded and up in the air
- Vintage clothes, which impart a sense of disharmony and lack of focus

ACCESSORIES

Position yourself for power with these awesome accessories.

Feng Shui Do's

- Frogs, for prosperity
- Sun, for leadership prowess
- Dragon, for the ultimate symbol of power (why do you think they called Leona Helmsley "the dragon lady"?)
- Flowers, for success
- Dogs, for protection
- Musical instruments, for concensus and power-building
- Crystals, for clarity and vision (Stevie Nicks gave us the heads up on this one in Fleetwood Mac's smash song, "Dreams")

Feng Shui Don'ts

- Broken arrows—they lead to broken dreams
- Leather collars, which indicate bondage
- Teddy bears are cuddly, but signify powerlessness
- An overabundance of chains (think Jackie Stallone here) keep you chained in and earthbound

Zangtra Mind Journal and Ritual

Maintaining optimal flow (chi) in your life is the cornerstone of creating power. Doing so helps you shed old ideas and ideals and enter a new time of awareness and truth in your life.

Before writing in your journal, I invite you to light a white or aqua candle and recite the following blessing:

As I light my feng shui candle
I become aware of the healing

power of nature's benevolent energies.
I, too, can choose to manifest change and transformation:
I choose to become part of the cycle of life.
I transcend separateness and dissolve into the energy and
*   power of life.*

As you write, keep the following issues in mind.
- Why am I seeking power?
- For what reasons do I call upon power in my life?
- How do I define power? (Remember, you need to be specific in order to create the kind of power you seek.)
- How can I use power for sources higher than myself, or for the public good?
- How will the power I bring into my life benefit my family and friends?

ZANGTRA EXERCISE
A short but effective yoga break is the perfect way to invite power into your life. This is because the dormant snake located at the root of your spine will arise and help you manifest new opportunities into your life. Today, there's a yoga center in nearly every nook and cranny of the United States and I can't recommend learning more about this ancient melding of spirit and fitness highly enough.

Here's the power zone zangtra exercise.
1. Stand up tall, and straighten your spine.
2. Place your feet apart and put the palm of your hand on the back of your waist, sliding midway to your buttocks. (This helps you lift your treasures upward.)
3. Pause for five seconds, then repeat.
Next . . .
4. Place your back against the wall with your feet apart, and bend your knees slightly.

5. Straighten the curve of your back as you gently ease your spine against the wall. Don't force it—let this happen naturally; this is called "opening the center door of life," and it beautifully readjusts your chi by strengthening your body's pagoda of power.

CHAPTER THIRTEEN

Fame: The Tiara Zone

KOAN
"Those who seek harmony know how to find it."

ZONE OM
"Be enlightened, and you will always find your way."

ZONE OM TIP
Place your zone om on the door of your bedroom closet to give yourself the recognition and self-esteem you deserve.

COLORS | Purple, red
SILHOUETTE | Triangle
BODY | Head

Zone Wisdom

In this zone, you will learn how to
- identify precisely the kind of recognition you seek
- gain the confidence required to sustain public recognition
- understand the difference between recognition by those you love and public acclaim

Zone Profile

Who among us hasn't secretly dreamed of being the "lady in red"? Whether we're the shy, retiring type or feel we were born to be a star, all of us seek at least a short time in the limelight.

However, before we can light our fires of fame, we have to be *present.* Call this focus, call it dedication, call it whatever you like. But always remember this: The recognition you seek, either in your personal or professional lives, doesn't come easy. For every Kate Moss, who was magically discovered waiting in line at an airport, there are a thousand women who had to work hard to get to the top. Women like:

- Madonna, who spent years learning to dance, write songs, and otherwise hone her craft (everyone who's ever met the former Material Girl says there's a reason she's a monster star: Madonna works harder than anyone else on the planet)
- Estée Lauder, who went salon to salon selling her products, laying the groundwork for one of the country's largest privately owned businesses
- Sally Ride, who earned a Ph.D. and trained for years before boarding that spaceship to the stars

Being present, keeping an eye on the prize, and grabbing the gold ring when the time is right is what this zone is all about. Until you learn to do just that, the fame and recognition you seek will remain an elusive and unattainable goal.

Feng shui associates this zone very closely with the five senses of touch, sight, hearing, taste, and smell. This is because only by using our tactile senses to the very fullest can we appreciate the world around us, and in so doing be present in every possible way. In simple parlance, it's about uncovering every stone—and not missing a single trick. If you look at people who are celebrated—whether their field be artistic, commercial, or not-for-profit—you will more often than not find this to be true. I love Woody Allen's famous quote that "80 percent of success is just showing up." And indeed, it's still surprising to me that so many people don't even show up— they're just not present in the most important parts of their lives.

The video store slacker has seeped into national pop culture as the most identifiable symbol of "non-presence." Now, there's nothing wrong with working in a video store. What's troublesome are the vacant eyes of kids who just don't care. If the video store job is a stepping-stone, that's perfect; if it's a virtual metaphor for a lack of goals, it ain't.

That said, it's up to you to make the most of this presence by keeping your eyes and ears open, and your wits about you. Only by using your God-given senses to the utmost can you seize the moment, capture the day, and take one more step on the road to the recognition that is rightfully yours.

At the same time, it's important to know what "the prize" is; as the saying goes, different strokes for different folks. We live, I'm sure you know, in a fame-obsessed society. Never has there been such a plethora of magazines, TV shows, and other media outlets devoted to the every movement of Brad and Jennifer, Matt and Ben. (Okay, I know they're not a couple, but they seem to be otherwise joined at the hip.) If Clooney chases a chick, we know about it; when Calista chews on a cookie, we all cheer. Once upon a time, there was only TV, but now there's cable, the Internet, satellite, and more—and each one needs to fill time and space with celebrity chatter.

All of which is fine, except for this: Our rabid national interest in celebrity sometimes seem to obscure more important values and concerns. Not everyone needs to be internationally famous or adored by millions of fans. For many folks, it's enough to be loved by our family and friends and to have the time and health to love them back. Or, on a professional plane, maybe we want to be recognized within our communities, throughout our state, or nationally within our fields.

That's where your zone om and koan come into play. We first need to seek enlightenment and harmony—to know who we are and our larger place in the universe—to fully reap the rewards of fame. This also allows us to set goals that are not only attainable, but right for us. As we said earlier, some folks may set their sights on global recognition, while for others it's enough to be the best baker in Bayonne, or the most marvelous mom in Montana.

By voicing our personal aims, we are able to focus on their attainment day in and day out. Specificity is key. I actually met a high school senior recently and asked what her goals were. "I want to be famous," she languidly replied. Well, honey, that's fine; so did Madonna, Estée, and Sally Ride. And despite their wildly disparate fields, they all did one thing: They defined the kind of recognition they sought, then went after it—with a vengeance, in every single case, and working their butts off all the while.

So can you, if you follow the Feng Shui Chic that follows. Whether you want your name up in lights or hanging on a shingle outside your front door, this is the chapter that will get you there.

Fashion Profile

You are a trailblazer in this all-eyes-on-you zone. This is where you are your most outgoing, vivacious, and courageous. Become a sun goddess, embrace the light—and soon *you'll* be the brightest star, whatever you do, wherever you live, whoever you are. Star Jones of ABC's *The View* is a marvelous example of this attitude. No shrinking violet, she wants to be princess of pizzazz, and always succeeds. Her mama knew what she was doing when she named her "Starlet"!

SILHOUETTE
An A-line is the look that helps you make a beeline for fame. Try a triangular wrap over straight pants . . . a '60's-style cone-shaped dress that flares out at the bottom . . . or an A-shaped coat over a short, straight skirt for recognition in all that you do.

The Face of Fame

Is it any surprise that the head and, of course, the face rule the fame zone? The tools to building a better reputation in your community, career, or even in Tinseltown can all be found in your makeup bag. Be sure your tools are in tip-top shape by regularly updating your bag and keeping all items sanitary and clean. A messy makeup bag reflects an unorganized mind, and while a fabulous face can take you far, an organized mind is more likely to bring the fame and fortune you deserve.

Lip Tips

Association	Lip shape	Color/finish
Creativity	Curved, elongated top lip	High sheen, pearlized, opalescent
	Regular lower lip	Blue or gray base
Power	Full upper lip	Berries, plums, peaches
	Thin lower lip	Beige or brown base
Action	Pointed peak top lip	Magenta, reds, pinks
	Regular lower lip	Pink, orange base
Balance	Arched top lip	Browns, terra cotta, brick, sienna
	Pouty lower lip	Yellow base
Wisdom	Elongated top lip	Silver, gold, copper, high shine
	Thin lower lip	White base

Eyebrow Tips

Association	Brow shape	Color
Creativity	Curved, elongated	Black, gray
Power	Full inner brow	Blond, ash tones
Action	High peaks, upward slant	Red-brown
Balance	Arcs, shortened line	Medium/dark brown
Wisdom	Thin/thick straight arc	Gray/silver, golden/copper, brown/blond

Feng Shui Do's

- Be a rodeo queen! A low-cut top paired with an oversized wrap makes you O.K. in any corral.
- Hot, trendy fashions put you on the inside track to fame.
- Dramatic designs, like a cheongsam (a traditional Chinese dress with a high slit to show off the leg), demand recognition from one and all.
- Off-the-shoulder tops tell the world you're ready to fly straight to the top.
- Halter tops let you stick your neck out toward the new opportunities you seek in this zone.
- For the office, a turtleneck coupled with an inverted-panel skirt show the world who's really the boss!

Feng Shui Don'ts

- Don't short-fuse your success by wearing a miniskirt at the office.
- You're a star, not an unsolved mystery—so avoid oversized out-

fits that hide who you really are. (I'm delighted to see that songstress Natalie Merchant has finally taken this advice. When she was with 10,000 Maniacs, she wore shapeless *schmattes;* on her *Motherland* CD cover, Miss M is wearing a tight, form-fitting top that literally shouts, "I'm a star!")

- Prim or powerful? It's up to you. If you button up like Snow White, you'll be drowning in dwarves—hardly a diva's delight.
- Flounces and ruffles keep you blowin' in the wind, not marching toward recognition and fame.

COLORS

The vibrant colors of this zone provide you with the power you need . . . on every step of the way to the recognition that is rightfully yours.

Feng Shui Do's

- Red, for an energy boost
- Purple, for devotion
- Orange, for health and personal attraction
- Yellow, to stimulate your intellect and provide strength

Feng Shui Don'ts

- White, which cools and drains passion from your soul
- Black, which overwhelms you and distracts you from your goals
- Brown, which imparts a stagnant energy

FABRICS

These fine fabrics feed your internal fire, lighting your road to recognition.

The Highlights of Your Life

If you want your name in lights, the highlights are your "mane" tool. Select the hair color, style, accessory shape, and color that best suits your goals as well as your fashion sense to gain the glory you seek. After all, you can't wear your tiara without the proper 'do.

Association	Hair color	Hair style	Accessory shape	Accessory color
Intuition	Black, with blue, green, or lavender hues	Loose, undefined, relaxed, wavy, uneven, curved	Curved, wavy, nautical	Black, indigo
Power	Golden blond, golden brown	Windblown, blunt cut, ponytail	Wood, square	Green
Sensuality	Red, red-brown, amber	Shag, pointed and layered, bangs, fringes	Stars, zigzags, jewels, sparkles	Red
Spirit	Ash brown, ash blond, charcoal, brown-black	Classic bun, French twist	Shells, flowers, minerals, animal prints	Yellow
Trendiness	Silver, gray, platinum blond with frosting and/or streaking	Wired, overcurled, spiked, parted sections	Metallics, rectangular shaped	White

- Satin, for power
- Metallics, for energy
- Brocade, to manifest ambition

Feng Shui Don'ts

- Leather, which shows you carrying your own baggage
- Netting, which portrays an inflated ego
- Corduroy, which interrupts intention and flow
- Mohair, which is fuzzy and unfocused

PATTERNS

Move over, modesty; enter the elaborate! The patterns you seek in this zone are fancy and fine—just what you'd expect from the face of fame.

Feng Shui Do's

- Pyramids, for power
- Animals, for basic instincts and expression (but avoid pigs, horses, teddy bears, eagles, deer, snakes, ants, butterflies, turtles, bees, flies, dogs, ladybugs, and kittens)
- Stars, because you are one
- Fruit, for fruitful endeavors, whatever they may be
- Sunbursts, for energy and light
- Birds, to give flight to all that you do

Feng Shui Don'ts

- Larger patterns, which portray you as an obstructionist
- Jagged patterns, which sever the ties that bind you to success
- Tie-dyes, which show a flaky, moving-in-circles you

ACCESSORIES

Bold, simple accessories ravishingly reflect your focus and intent. Wear them liberally in the recognition zone.

Feng Shui Do's

- Charm bracelets, for social contacts
- Triangles, for power
- Red roses, for growth
- Trees, for power and stature
- Gold boat, to show your ship has come in
- Tiaras and laurel crowns, for the ultimate recognition—your self-coronation!

Feng Shui Don'ts

- Angels—you want to be earthbound, not up in the air
- Raindrops, which put out your passion and fire

Zangtra Mind Journal and Ritual

To clear your path to fame, place a purple candle nearby and recite or meditate upon this blessing:

*As I light this flame, I focus on receiving
I choose to participate fully in the game of life*

Becoming healthy and vibrant in the process
As I embrace the winds of the sky and the waters of the
earth
I become part of the perpetual flow and exchange of Yin
and Yang energies
When my pulse dances with nature, I find harmony
When my spirit embraces polarity, I find balance
Unless there is an opposing wind, a kite cannot fly
I meditate on the riddle, seeking enlightenment
A single intuitive spark fuels the fire of understanding
I reach for new heights and new challenges, and
I celebrate the joy of success

After reciting or meditating on this blessing, I ask you to consider the following questions as you journal.

- What is bothering me most right now and keeping me from the fame that I seek?
- What, specifically, are my goals? Be very precise, because only then can you achieve them. For instance:
  1. "I want to be the hottest haircutter in Hartford."
  2. "I seek a recording contract and to have my music known all around the world."
  3. "I'd like my husband to recognize all the work that I do for our family."

Remember, this is the zone of both fame and recognition, and these can mean very different things to different people. Also keep in mind that this is all about attaining the kind of recognition you seek for yourself—not the road your parents, friends, or teachers may have mapped for you.

- What gives me the most confidence; what am I best at? When we ask ourselves this question, we can identify our most powerful self—our first foot forward on the road to recognition.

Reading Your Glasses

If the eyes are the windows to our soul, then our eyeglasses are the windowframes. How you choose to decorate your frames reveals a great deal about your spirit as well as your style.

Association	Frame shape	Frame color/Pattern	Glass tint
Intelligence	Oval	Black, blue, tortoise, opalescent, pearlized, shells, faux stone	Mirror, blue, black
Power	Square	Green, bamboo, rattan, teak, jungle print, silk finish	Green, aqua, UV ray
Sensuality	Peaked, elongated	Red, pink, purple, animal prints	Pink, lavender
Spirit	Square, round	Brown, yellow, floral, camouflage, reptile	Amber, brown, yellow
Trendiness	Rectangle	White, metallic, plastic, animal patterns	Gray, amber, rose

ZANGTRA EXERCISE

Tao teaches us that our eyes are the windows of our souls. Moreover, our eyes can help us to develop positive chi by keeping an eye on our wellness and health. Think of this like adjusting the tracking on your VCR.

Perform this exercise by following these steps:

1. Keep your eyes open and visualize a T in your mind.
2. Center the T in the middle of your forehead. Is it slightly off the mark? If so, slowly bring the T to the very center of your forehead.

Another good way to go is this way . . .

Fame: The Tiara Zone | **187**

1. Rotate your eyes clockwise while keeping your head still.
2. Slowly move your eyes to the ceiling, then right, then back to the center; then to the left, then back to the ceiling.
3. Repeat nine times.
4. Now, do the same exercise ten times in a counterclockwise fashion.

By performing this exercise several times a day, you will begin to feel centered and at peace—in a perfect place to start creating the power to make important changes in your life.

CHAPTER FOURTEEN

Nurture: The Good

Works Zone

KOAN
"Gems are polished by rubbing, just as man is made brilliant by trials."

ZONE OM
"What lies underneath is for you to discover."

ZONE OM TIP
Place your zone om in your kitchen or on the door of your pantry or refrigerator to receive the abundance of the universe in the nurture zone.

COLORS | Yellow, brick
SILHOUETTE | Square, rectangle
BODY | Stomach, spleen

Zone Wisdom

In this zone, you will learn how to
- recognize the core essence of your true nature
- hear your own personal melody and love your own, unique life
- dance to your life's music . . . and, in so doing, nurture your spirit and soul

- invite the rest of the world into your joyous dance—especially those whom you hold most dear

Zone Profile

We come, gentle reader, to the ultimate zone chapter in this book. Just as I celebrate coming to this point—for it is, in many ways, the culmination of my own life's work—so too do I joyously welcome you to the nurture zone.

Why is this so? Because when all is said and done, our joy in life is in many ways the direct result of how well we treat ourselves: how we love and nurture our heart and soul. This zone is the sweet synthesis of all the other zones, and of our whole life experience; it is the area of abundance and amplitude, of our own vision and voice.

Why abundance? Because we want to fill our bodies and souls with an open acceptance of the universe and of all God's gifts. This is always the very first step to nurturing our spirits—not only in this zone, but through all the days of our lives. So, in short: Open yourself to receiving all the power and possibilities from within and without. Feel the wisdom, joy, and very life force that resides not only in the world outside but deep within yourself.

Indeed, this openness leads not only to personal empowerment, but to the healing forces that will make your life healthy and grand. It's no wonder at all that this zone is associated with the stomach, where our solar plexus is located, and the spleen, which cleanses our bodies of bile, which we can make a conscious effort to replace with beauty and bounty in all that we do.

Once we purify ourselves spiritually and physically, we can begin to discover the essence of who we are. This is what our zone om tells us: By finding what lies underneath, we come to the core and can learn precisely who we are, and about those things that mean the most to us.

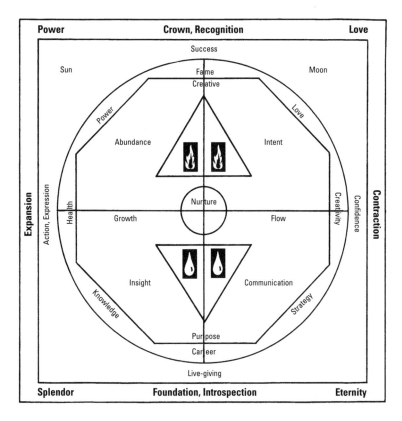

Power	**Crown, Recognition**	**Love**

Success

Sun | Fame | Moon
Creative

Power | | Love

Abundance | | Intent

Nurture

Growth | | Flow

Insight | | Communication

Knowledge | | Strategy

Purpose
Career

Live-giving

Splendor	**Foundation, Introspection**	**Eternity**

Expansion · Action, Expression · Health

Contraction · Creativity · Confidence

Energy Map

How can we do this? By listening to the music of our very own lives. As the saying goes, we all march to our own drummer, and only when we find the tunes he is beating along to can we find our best, truest, and most joyous self.

According to Traditional Chinese Medicine (TCM), our stomach is our "internal bagpipe"; that's why this area of the body is tied to this zone. What's more, TCM tells us that our lungs are our body's lute, because our lungs breathe air that regulates our body's chi.

Nurture: The Good Works Zone | **191**

The fire energy of our upper body and water energy of our lower torsos come together just below our stomachs, at the solar plexus. When their alignment is perfect, we are as one—altogether whole in positive forward movement, and in every way an awesome force to be reckoned with! It is at this time, when we feel most at peace, that our body is a fine-tuned musical instrument, producing lute-like tones of joy and peace.

You also know, from way back in chapter three, how feng shui is inextricably tied to the environment and to the greater world in which we live. Nowhere is this more apparent than in the nurture zone. I invite you to step outside and hear nature's voices sing; as you do, you will begin to appreciate—and, I hope, come to love—the healing harmonics of Planet Earth.

Listen to the symphonies of grass sighing, and to the soft caress as entire meadows embrace the wind. Even in a crowded city, you can hear (if the time is right!) the rustling of the leaves on trees. There's a lesson to be learned here: The sound of nature in all her glory teaches us to blow with the breeze, to go with the flow. Watch the leaves blow and let your own personal flag of joy unfurl as well.

Nature's harmony is as figurative as it is audible. Just think of it: The leaves change color, new blooms bud, and the world is blanketed with sunshine or snow as the seasons parade before us. And just as nature changes, so too must we embrace change, which helps us create new directions for personal harmony and inner growth. It is this theme, friends, that best defines the nurture zone.

Finally, this is the zone to come to when all else seems to fail. I don't care who you are—a woman of fortune, an average American, or the proverbial maid of constant sorrow. We all have ups and downs in our lives: hills to climb, valleys to climb out of, and beautiful vistas to enjoy once we have ascended to our perfect places. I pray that all of us might know more delight than dismay; but I know, too, that we all have moments of madness and pain, times when nothing seems right.

Remember Natalie Imbruglia's song "Torn"? It was a monster hit not only in this country and Natalie's native Australia, but all around the world. In addition to a stirring melody—and you know how important music is in this zone—it conveyed a sentiment that touched millions of people's lives: What to do at those times when nothing seems to fit, when you, like the song's heroine, are lying naked on the floor—when, in fact, you are nothing less than "torn"?

That's exactly when you should follow the steps I outline in this zone. This is where you come when you need to set things straight, fine-tune your spirits, and ask your battered soul to help you fly higher and prouder than you ever did before.

And you will, my dears, you will; the advice I provide in this chapter will teach you exactly how.

NURTURING SCENTS

In chapter four, I shared the best scents for your element type. But because this is the zone of taking care of yourself, I'm happy to share these outcome-specific scents to lift your spirits whenever you like.

- Angelica, for concentration
- Basil, to clarify
- Cedar, to cleanse
- Chamomile, to calm
- Fennel, to relax
- Geranium, for harmony
- Lavender, to soothe
- Lemon, to uplift
- Lime, to invigorate
- Orange, for sweetness
- Patchouli, for sensuality
- Peony, for beauty
- Pine, for longevity
- Rose, for emotional uplift
- Rosemary, for focus
- Sage, to cleanse
- Sandalwood, for sensuality
- Thyme, to stimulate

As you do so, in this final and most important zone, I wish you all the luck and love in the world.

Fashion Profile

No one typifies the nurture zone more fully and fabulously than the late, great Diana, Princess of Wales.

Every book that you read about Diana, every interview with a friend, returns to the same place: Princess Diana's sons were her life. She may have tripped up from time to time in other areas, but when it came to princes William and Harry, Diana was a royal success.

Of course, that was just the beginning for this remarkable woman. Once a shy, unsure teen, she was determined to become a woman of substance. How did she do it? After bouts of depression and anorexia, Princess Diana decided to nurture herself—and, in so doing, she nurtured everyone around her as well. That, I think, is the greatest lesson of her lovely life.

Many royals or celebrities are shockingly self-obsessed. Not Diana, whose charity work became the very touchstone of her life. No royal had ever touched AIDS patients; she did. They had certainly not embraced young African war victims; she did. And they had certainly never traipsed across land mines in an effort to rid the world of these hideous traps; she did. Princess Diana was the very essence of the nurture zone—not because of her beauty or her glamour, but because of her gracious, nurturing good works. We don't think of outlandish outfits or cheap costumes when it comes to this definitive class act. What we do think of is a look in which comfortable chic rules. But beware: Comfortable doesn't mean messy, disheveled, or otherwise out to lunch, but a look that lets you, not your clothes, take charge. Here, showing off isn't the score. Instead, you've got to be free to nurture yourself and others—and that's exactly what this zone's style stance is all about.

Many folks mistakenly feel that fashion is frivolous, fluffy, and self-involved. Not so! While it is true that we have all known souls—women and men alike—who are all style and no substance, there is absolutely nothing wrong with acknowledging the importance of fashion in our lives. The ancients knew this and used their version of Feng Shui Chic to influence outcomes in their lives—and so, too, can you.

Finally, please respect this indisputable fact: By using fashion wisely, you are respecting yourself. Even more than that, you are nurturing yourself—and that, after all, is what this chapter is all about.

SILHOUETTE

Sleek and slender is your silhouette salvo for the nurture zone. This feng shui silhouette does double duty by keeping you anchored to the ground while showing you to be upward and onward in all that you do.

Feng Shui Do's

- Long coats paint you as tailored and sleek, while still giving you the freedom to nurture all in your world
- Cargo pants combine natural comfort with fashion flair
- A fitted jacket with slim (not cigarette) pants suits you for success in the nurture zone. It shows you to be kindly in control and ready to nurture everyone and everything in your life.
- For nifty nurture on the home front, become a caftan queen. But take note: Here, I'm advising a long, straight Moroccan djellaba–type garment, not a Mama Cass–like caftan that could span the Atlantic and back!

Feng Shui Don'ts

- Never tie yourself up with laces and straps. These restrict your growth and keep you bound in. How could you possibly nurture anyone or anything in this state?
- Leave the tornadoes in Kansas and hurricanes in Haiti! Large, circular, flowing skirts or gowns create sails, which are bad for business or personal occasions—in either case, you'll be passed over in a whirlwind.
- Reject the ruffles, especially on an important date. These tell your beau (or belle, if Ellen DeGeneres does more for you than Brad Pitt) that you've got too much steam, and not enough passionate heat.
- Structured ensembles are the very opposite of what zings in this zone. Instead, let your body wake up to the nurturing forces of nature with less rigid (though remember, never sloppy) silhouettes.

COLORS

Think of the calming colors of the nurture zone as your palette of harmony. These earthy colors help connect you to Mother Earth and let you become a Nurture Queen of note.

Feng Shui Do's

- Yellow, for bright sunshine and good cheer (Note: ocher and goldenrod are especially good tones here.)
- Orange, for the power to nurture all you hold dear
- Peach, for its nurturing effect on friendships
- Metallics, to unblock your personal passion for relationships and love

- Red, which makes you dusty, dry, and devoid of nurturing energy
- Black, especially when combined with brown—it drains you of energy and love
- Blue, especially when worn with black—this paints you as bruised, the very opposite of the nurturing forces you seek

FABRICS

As with silhouette, comfort is key here. In this zone, always choose fabrics that are soft, flexible, and breathe (and that let *you* breathe). Leave the spandex in your closet—the big news is natural fabrics in this very important zone.

Feng Shui Do's

- Denim, which lets you get down to basics
- Cotton, which puts you in touch with nature
- Silk, which smoothes your way to nurturing bliss
- Flannel, for the comfort you need to nurture others—and yourself

Feng Shui Don'ts

- Cracked or scruffy fabrics, which promote disharmony
- Patches of any kind. Anne Tyler may call it *A Patchwork Planet,* but I don't—very bad feng shui in this zone
- Netting, which puts you up in the clouds—a million miles away from the sure-footed grounding you need here

PATTERNS
In this zone, the patterns you wear should reflect Earth's rapidly changing patterns. This roots you to the healing and nurturing forces of the natural world.

Feng Shui Do's

- Paisleys, for expansion
- Plaids, for prosperity
- Fruit, for fertility
- Animals, for instinctive nurture
- Flowers, to promote new opportunities

Feng Shui Don'ts

- X's, which cross yourself out. You're alive and kicking, not dead and gone!
- Clouds and stars, which portray you as up in the air—not grounded, as you need to be here
- Nautical symbols, which show you as unanchored and out to sea
- Camouflage prints, which hide you from all whom you love

ACCESSORIES
Your goal here is to use accessories that boost your energy. In so doing, you can harness the power you need to bestow nurturing energy throughout every aspect of your life.

Feng Shui Do's

- Flowered scarves let you commune with nature and seed new opportunities everywhere you go.
- Gold tones bring nurturing sun energy to all that you do and to everyone you meet.

- Copper bracelets provide healing energy to your body; this lets you nurture other folks as well.
- Charms express your affection for all living things.
- Angels and fairies keep you out of harm's way.
- Grapes give your life sweetness and joy.
- Lions are your guardians, protecting the nurturing energy in your life.
- Cranes and swans are associated with longevity—perfect in this zone.
- Bells show that you respect all life on Earth.
- Butterflies make you jump for joy and let you infect others with your raging good cheer.

Feng Shui Don'ts

- Lizards promote fear, not the nurturing attitude you want.
- Downward-pointing elephant trunks drain your energy and health.
- Safety pins (sorry, Vivienne Westwood!) show that your soul needs mending, the very opposite of what you seek in this zone.

Zangtra Mind Journal and Ritual

Before beginning your zangtra activities, please light an amber-colored candle. This provides protection and fosters the nurturing energy within you.

Recite the following blessing:

> *I call upon the chi energy of the Earth, asking that the animals of the Earth be blessed, strengthened, and protected. I honor my connectedness with all of the earth's species. I welcome protection, security, and peace for myself, my home, and for the planet.*

Nurture: The Good Works Zone | **199**

Your zangtra diary in the nurture zone is nothing short of a golden opportunity. It allows you to think about every aspect of your life and to journal your hopes, fears, and dreams in their largest, most universal context.

Remember, as I said in the beginning of this chapter, that this is one that ties all the other zones together. Focus your mind, and as you write, think about these questions.

- What can I do to make myself more grounded?
- How can I spend time to nurture my own soul, as a prerequisite to nurturing others?
- How can I give back to Earth and to my fellow travelers through life?
- What are some of the things I do that are non-nurturing to my body and soul?

and, finally

- Who in my life most needs my nurturing love right now, and how can I help them?
- What can I do to use the nurturing energy the universe has provided me with to best help people on both local and global levels? How can I promote love, healing, and wonder in all that I do?

I have one special secret that I'd especially like to share with you. As a prelude to asking myself these questions—and yes, readers, I do practice what I preach—I like to take a long hike. In addition to being my absolute favorite kind of exercise, hiking has a very specific connection to the nurture zone: It allows us to physically connect with Mother Earth and gain her guidance, practically via osmosis, as we consider the big questions of the nurture zone. (In fact, some of my clients like to hike before journaling in any zone, as it clears their heads and reminds them of the glory of the natural world; this is especially so if we walk in the mountains, across a flowered meadow, or in any other place of beauty and peace.)

An affirmation of which I am very fond:

I stand with my body planted
solidly upon the earth,
and the Spiritual light of Heaven
fills my heart and
illuminates my spirit and path.
By illuminating my pathway,
I help to manifest harmony
and balance in my life,
and create heaven on Earth.

Reciting or reading this affirmation as you finish your hike and just before you start your journaling helps focus your mind and lets you revel in the thought patterns that will provide answers to your questions and illuminate you on your way.

ZANGTRA EXERCISE

Just as a tree roots in the ground for its balance and nurture, this zangtra exercise will allow you to connect to Mother Earth for the nurture you need in every part of your life. To do this exercise, follow these steps.

1. Stand straight, sinking down to the ground as comfortably as you can with slightly separated knees.
2. Raise your arms, bringing them forward slightly above your waist. Imagine that you are embracing a tree as you do.
3. Turn your toes slightly inward, as if you were on a saddle. As you sink downward into your knees, you will feel the connection between your knees and ankles. Feel your body as a force that is passing from your own bone structure downward to the ground.
4. Press downward, turning your knees outward; feel yourself a root connecting to the earth.
5. Feel this energy and align yourself spiritually with the earth; this allows you to increase your inner strength.

NATURE'S OWN
NURTURE

There are those who call jewels ostentatious, gaudy, and in your face. Honey, I say the Hope Diamond is one trinket I'd love to call my own!

Seriously, why be ashamed of sporting a gem? They are nature's own bounty, and ours to enjoy. Better still is that feng shui associates certain gems with specific outcomes in the nurture zone. Glitter and glean good things with these gems below.

- Tigereye and jasper, for nurture
- Cinnabar and amber, for desire
- Citrine and yellow moonstone, for power
- Pink tourmaline and jade, for love
- Lapis, turquoise, and aquamarine, for communication skills
- Amethyst, for heightened spirit and introspection

continued on next page

6. Do this exercise six times at first, building to twelve repetitions as you progress.

Let me give you a good example of how one of my clients used this exercise to wonderful effect. Joie is one of those people who, on the outside, was always cheerful and upbeat. Her whole life was devoted to fulfilling the wishes of others, rather than acknowledging and respecting her own needs. In sum, she was nurturing everyone else in her world except the one who mattered most—herself.

Instead, Joie took on the weight of the world, or at least her immediate world, by taking on the concerns of everyone else. In a sense, she sought to make herself indispensable—and thus important and liked—but what she ended up doing was ignoring her own body and mind. Along the way, Joie put on about twenty pounds, which I believe to be a physical manifestation of her inner struggle.

Joie was a perfect candidate for the steps I outline in this, the nurture chapter. Given the manifestation of issues in her body—the increase in weight—I advised her to start with the zangtra exercise. I reasoned that, by allowing Joie to connect with the earth, she would be making important first steps in connecting with her own needs. In a sense, she would be nurturing herself by harnessing the power of Mother Earth.

- Clear quartz, for clarity
- Garnet, for focus
- Diamond, for eternal love
- Emerald, for healing
- Pearl, for love
- Sapphire, for rejuvenation
- Jade, for protectoin
- Turquoise, for friendship

That was precisely what Joie did. This exercise put her very much in touch with her body; and by journaling, asking herself the questions we posed in the mind journal section above, she was able to "make the connection" between her issues of spirit and self. The next week, Joie began by following the fashion advice in the first part of the chapter. After only a few weeks, I am glad to report that, by acknowledging herself and nurturing her own needs, Joie began to lose weight and started to put herself first. Today, several years later, she looks and feels like the super person she is.

A Fond Farewell

to You . . . and a

Happy Hello to

Feng Shui Chic

There, dear friends, you have it—the beautiful basics of Feng Shui Chic. I hope you will use the knowledge you have gained in this book now . . . and forever.

In the very first chapter, I promised that I'd share with you my life's work, and that I have done. Over the past three decades, I have amassed my own knowledge of the classic art of feng shui and melded it to fit modern times. In these pages, I have shared my joyous knowledge of feng shui in the hope that you will use this information to make your life the best and most joyous one you can.

One last time, I ask you to recall that the practice of feng shui is a three-tiered art, one that incorporates mind, body, and spirit. I know how attractive easy fixes can be—wear red, and you'll find love; tie on a green bow, and money will flow your way—but remember that this is only part of the story. If we don't acknowledge the spiritual aspect of feng shui or its mind–body connection, we will not enjoy the fullest benefits it can impart to our lives.

For that reason, I ask you to use every section of any given chapter to the fullest. If, for example, your focus is on fame, it is not enough to wear the colors, fabrics, or fashion silhouette I prescribe. You must solicit the power of your own mind and thoughtforms by stating your intent, then cementing your intent by diligently writing in your journal and performing your zangtra exercises in concert with each other. For maximal effect, I invite my friends and clients to think of feng shui as a team sport involving your body, mind, and soul. I sincerely hope you will do the very same.

Above all, remember this: The decision to influence outcomes in your life is yours and yours alone. By acknowledging the energies of colors, fabrics, and gems—and even the power of the foods you eat—you can be the mistress of your world . . . now, tomorrow, and in all the days to come. In the end, it is you who creates the positive energy and joy every day that you live.

There are days when we feel all Earth's blessings—when we are in perfect alignment with nature, the world, and our own selves. The bounty of the universe is yours if you just ask for it . . . and you can help it along with a little bit of Feng Shui Chic. By unleashing the power of feng shui, you can attain your most cherished dreams: at home, at work, and in every aspect of your life. I wish you nothing less than joy, health, and happiness—plus all the spirit and style!—in the world.

Blessings and light,
Carole Swann Meltzer
New York City

RESOURCES

FENG SHUI

Carter, Karen Rauch. *Move Your Stuff, Change Your Life: How to Use Feng Shui to Get Love, Money, Respect, and Happiness.* New York: Simon & Schuster, 2000.

Collins, Terah Kathryn. *Home Design with Feng Shui, A–Z.* Carlsbad, CA: Hay House, 1999.

———. *The Western Guide to Feng Shui: Creating Balance, Harmony, and Prosperity in Your Environment.* Carlsbad, CA: Hay House, 1996.

———. *The Western Guide to Feng Shui for Prosperity.* Carlsbad, CA: Hay House, 2002.

———. *The Western Guide to Feng Shui, Room by Room.* Carlsbad, CA: Hay House, 1999.

Kennedy, David Daniel. *Feng Shui for Dummies.* Foster City, CA: IDG Books Worldwide, 2001.

Kingston, Karen. *Clear Your Clutter with Feng Shui.* New York: Broadway Books, 1999.

Rossbach, Sarah, and Master Lin Yun. *Feng Shui Design: From History and Landscape to Modern Gardens and Interiors.* New York: Viking, 1998.

Sang, Larry. *The Principles of Feng Shui.* Monterey Park, CA: American Feng Shui Institute, 1994.

Shurety, Sarah. *Quick Feng Shui Cures: Simple Solutions and Secret Tips for a Healthy, Happy, and Successful Life.* New York: Hearst Books, 1999.

Skinner, Stephen. *Living Earth Manual of Feng Shui: Chinese Geomancy.* London: Arkana, 1989.

CHINESE CULTURE

Beijing College of Traditional Chinese Medicine. *Essential Chinese Acupuncture.* Beijing: Foreign Language Press, 1980.

Chen Huoping. *Fun with Chinese Characters.* Straits Times Collection. Singapore: Federal Publications, 1980.

Cleary, Thomas. *The Taoist Classics,* vol. I. Boston: Shambhala, 1999.

Fahr-Becker, Gabriele, ed. *The Art of East Asia.* Cologne: Konemann, 1998.

Foo, Lillian. *Chinese Numerology in Feng Shui.* Kuala Lumpur: Konsep Books, 1994.

Gombrich, E. M. *Art and Illusion: A Study in the Psychology of Pictorial Representation.* New York: Pantheon for Bollingen Foundation, 1960.

The I Ching, or Book of Changes. 3rd ed. The Richard Wilhelm Translation rendered into English by Cary F. Baynes. London: Routledge and Kegan Paul, 1968.

Kwan, Lau. *Secrets of Chinese Astrology: A Handbook of Self-Discovery.* New York: Tengu Books, 1994.

Kwok, Man-Ho. *Chinese Astrology.* Edited by Joanne O'Brien. Boston: E.C. Tuttle, 1997.

Lau, Kwan. *Secrets of Chinese Astrology.* New York: Tengu Books, 1994.

Li Zehou. *The Path of Beauty: A Study of Chinese Aesthetics.* Beijing: Morning Glory Publishers, 1988.

Lo, Eileen Yin-Fei. *Chinese Kitchen: Recipes, Techniques and Ingredients, History and Memories from America's Leading Authority on Chinese Cooking.* New York: Morrow, 1999.

Maoshing Ni. *The Yellow Emperor's Classic of Medicine: A New Translation of the Neijing Suwe.* Boston: Shambhala, 1995.

Walters, Derek. *Chinese Astrology: Interpreting the Revelations of the Celestial Messengers.* Wellingborough, Northamptonshire:

Aquarian Press; New York, NY: Distributed by Sterling Pub. Co., 1987.

Young, Grace. *The Wisdom of the Chinese Kitchen: Classic Family Recipes for Celebration and Healing.* New York: Simon & Schuster, 1999.

Zhao, Feng. *Treasures in Silk: An Illustrated History of Chinese Textiles.* Hangzhou, 1999.

OTHER

Battersby, Martin. *The Decorative Twenties.* New York: Whitney Library of Design, 1988.

———. *The Decorative Thirties.* New York: Whitney Library of Design, 1988.

Betty, Patricia, and David Andrusia. *Essential Beauty: Using Nature's Essential Oils to Rejuvenate, Replenish, and Revitalize.* Los Angeles: Keats Publishing, 2000.

Colbin, Annemarie. *Food and Healing.* New York: Ballantine Books, 1996.

Robbins, John. *Diet for New America.* Tiburon, CA: H. J. Kramer, 1998.

Rose, Jeanne. *Herbs and Things: Jeanne Rose's Herbal.* New York: Perigee, 1973.

Spiro, Audrey. *Contemplating the Ancients.* Berkeley, CA: University of California Press, 1990.

Tierra, Michael. *Planetary Herbology.* Twin Lakes, WI: Lotus Press, 1988.

The information in this book is derived from formulas and "trade secrets" translated by Grand Master Leung—my feng shui master and grand teacher of feng shui tenets. These translations have been handed to me in accordance with a master feng shui traditional ceremony in Hong Kong. These sacred texts are the translations from the original ancient silk manuscripts from Master

Leung's private collection. The original manuscripts are currently housed in the private collection at the Arthur Sakler Museum in Washington, D.C.

In accordance to the tradition of receiving the title master, I have incorporated these "trade secrets" to enhance and empower energy and promote healing and harmony for today's lifestyle.

Living well is an art.

Living in harmony with your environment is
Feng Shui Spirit.

Feng Shui Master Carole Swann Meltzer, B.T.B., has designed a wide range of Feng Shui Chic fashion, body-care, lifestyle, and home/office products to help you create the life you want to lead. Enhance creativity, gain clarity, and nurture harmony with these Feng Shui Spirit products:

- Chi-Om bracelets and necklaces
- Scented meditation and travel candles
- Spa body-care lotions, massage oils, and soaps
- Sage wands
- Harmony bowls
- Dream catchers
- Tabletop accessories
- and much more!

Also available are Feng Shui consultation services, including interior design consultation for home or office, and lifestyle coaching. To purchase these life-affirming products and/or arrange for a Feng Shui consultation, we welcome you to visit: **www.fengshuispirit.com.**